FACING
the UNSEEN

ALSO BY DAMON TWEEDY, M.D.

Black Man in a White Coat

FACING
the UNSEEN

THE STRUGGLE TO
CENTER MENTAL HEALTH
IN MEDICINE

DAMON TWEEDY, M.D.

ST. MARTIN'S
PRESS
NEW YORK

First published in the United States by St. Martin's Press, an imprint
of St. Martin's Publishing Group

FACING THE UNSEEN. Copyright © 2024 by Damon Tweedy.
All rights reserved. Printed in the United States of America.
For information, address St. Martin's Publishing Group,
120 Broadway, New York, NY 10271.

www.stmartins.com

The Library of Congress Cataloging-in-Publication Data
is available upon request.

ISBN 978-1-250-28489-1 (hardcover)

ISBN 978-1-250-28488-4 (ebook)

Our books may be purchased in bulk for promotional, educational, or
business use. Please contact your local bookseller or the Macmillan
Corporate and Premium Sales Department at 1-800-221-7945, extension
5442, or by email at MacmillanSpecialMarkets@macmillan.com.

First Edition: 2024

10   9   8   7   6   5   4   3   2   1

CONTENTS

AUTHOR'S NOTE

This book is based on my twenty-five years working at the intersection of general medicine and psychiatric care, first as a medical student, then as a medical intern, as a psychiatry resident, and finally, as a fully accredited psychiatrist. Names and other identifying details of patients have been changed, and in some cases, merged, to protect individual privacy. The same is true for the nurses, doctors, and other medical staff who cared for the patients described. In preparation for this manuscript, I spoke with more than a dozen people, locally and nationally, who have graciously consented to have their insights included herein. They are identified by professional title and their full names.

Although I have decades of accumulated knowledge on the subject, the crux of what follows is formed by my personal narrative, which means it can't possibly claim to speak for every facet of the mental health landscape. For starters, my entire professional medical career has taken place in one state, all within a one-hour radius of Duke University, where I attended medical school and completed my residency training. My work in psychiatry has mainly been in academic and government settings, with just a small amount in the private world.

On the latter note, there might be more variability between what one psychiatrist does compared with the next psychiatrist than in any medical discipline. Some of us work exclusively in private practice and offer psychotherapy only to self-paying clients. Others spend our days in jails and prisons, where we prescribe medications or conduct forensic evaluations.

Many combine psychotherapy and medication treatments. Still another cohort works in the growing field of electrical modulation of the brain. And a considerable number of us don't see patients at all but instead spend our professional lives as full-time researchers, educators, or health care administrators. No writing by a single psychiatrist could fully represent all these diverse perspectives.

It must also be said that psychiatrists are but one type of mental health professional. Psychologists, social workers, licensed professional counselors, marriage and family therapists, nurse practitioners, and physician assistants all independently see patients seeking mental health treatment. So do family physicians, gynecologists, emergency physicians, general internists, pediatricians, and an assortment of other medical doctors who were primarily trained to tend to the physical body. And while nurses are not licensed independent providers, they too are vital to the delivery of mental health services. The viewpoints of these nonpsychiatrist health care workers are essential to any discussion on mental health.

Finally, this book is not intended to dispense medical advice to individuals. Please consult with your health care providers, whether they are in general medicine, specialty practice, or the mental health care realm, before making decisions to change your current plan of care. Ultimately, it is this genuine exchange between a patient and the physician or other health care worker that will always be the foundation of good medicine, and no book can hope to substitute for that ancient tradition.

FACING

the UNSEEN

INTRODUCTION

ONE EARLY AFTERNOON SOME YEARS AGO WHILE WORKING IN A mental health clinic near a local jail and homeless shelter, I got a stomach-churning reminder of how much psychiatry differed from other medical specialties.

I had just sat down for a quick lunch at my cluttered desk when a nurse transferred a call from the primary care clinic located fifteen minutes away. I picked up the phone and heard the voice of Dr. Davis, a younger doctor in our system I'd met once months before. She started off talking fast. No hellos. No pleasantries. Straight to the point.

"This patient needs to see one of you guys," she said, her voice bordering on frantic. "He was going to shoot himself last week. He put a loaded handgun in his mouth, but his nine-year-old granddaughter walked in the room and stopped him."

For Dr. Davis to call me during lunch, rather than submit a mental health consult through our electronic system, I knew the situation was urgent in her mind. Initially, I assumed the patient was followed by one of my colleagues who was off duty that day, or on vacation. But this man wasn't seeing a psychiatrist, psychologist, or any mental health professional. Only Dr. Davis, a general physician whose training had focused on health problems like diabetes and pneumonia. Not suicide.

"Is he still thinking about shooting himself?" I asked. "Does he need to go to the hospital?"

"I told him about the psych ER," she said. "But he won't go."

Most people associate emergency rooms with heart attacks, gunshot wounds, appendicitis, and other medical-sounding problems. I didn't even know someone could go to a hospital emergency department for psychiatric reasons until my second year of medical school.

"Said he feels better now," she continued. "But he's been depressed for years, so I know he'll start feeling bad again. Can you help me persuade him to go? Can you see him?"

Months earlier, I'd ended a three-year stint taking ER shifts on Wednesday evenings. And the year before, I'd stopped working weekends at a private psychiatric hospital. I was settling into the more predictable life of an outpatient psychiatrist, where patients arrived at the clinic on their own and departed freely. No police. No locked units. Less drama.

"I still think you should call one of the emergency department psychiatric staff to see what they say," I told her. "I have patients all afternoon who've been scheduled for months."

Dr. Davis told me she'd spoken with a social worker and a psychiatry resident there but found neither helpful. She then complimented me on a mutual patient we shared and how I'd helped that person through a difficult time. Like many people, doctors included, I was a pushover for flattery, even if it added to my work. I looked at my watch. If the patient could get there in twenty minutes, maybe I could figure out a way to see him.

"Is he still with you now?" I asked.

"No. He said he had to pick up his granddaughter early from school. He said anything that kept him from getting her would only make things worse. So I told him I'd call him this afternoon with a plan. But it would be a lot better if you called him. You're the expert."

"How did this topic come up?" I asked, my approach methodical. "Did he offer up this information on his own, or did you ask him specific questions about suicide?"

In the moment, all I could think of were a series of questions to help me assist Dr. Davis as quickly as possible. The visceral human tragedy she described eluded me. It was only later that I thought about how my older son was just a few years younger than the child she'd mentioned. What would it have been like for him to walk in on my dad holding a gun to his head? And for my dad to have his grandson see him like that?

Had I been numbed by all the years of suffering I'd seen inside hospitals and clinics? Or, by focusing on assessment and triage, was I responding the way any decent psychiatrist would in this situation? By that point in my career, I increasingly found myself uncertain about the balance between being caring and being competent, and whether I could be both at the same time.

"I asked him if he'd ever been suicidal," Dr. Davis replied. "You know, for that depression screen we're supposed to do, though you guys should be the ones doing it. And he told me the story. He said at first he wasn't going to, but decided he didn't want to lie."

"What happened after the granddaughter found him?" I asked.

"He changed his mind," she said. "He gave his gun to his son and told him he didn't need it anymore. He said he hasn't had any thoughts about suicide since."

The general public continues to link gun violence with mass shooters, street gangs, and jealous boyfriends and husbands, but most shooting deaths, year after year, are self-inflicted. Especially in older men.

"Can you call him and sort this out?" Dr. Davis asked.

I understood how the emergency room social worker and psychiatrist didn't think this was an emergency: a week was an eternity from their perspectives. Still, I could see why Dr. Davis was so alarmed. It wasn't every day, at least not in *her* world, that a patient told her he'd recently come within minutes of shooting himself. Was he better now, a week later? Had he *really* gotten rid of all his guns?

"I'm not sure I should do that," I said hesitantly. "He doesn't know me at all. It would be weird for him to have me call out of the blue and start talking about suicide."

"If I tell him you're calling, he'll talk to you. This really shouldn't be my job. I'm supposed to be treating diabetes and high blood pressure. Not complex mental health stuff."

She made it sound as if there was a clear distinction between those who had kidney failure and heart disease on one hand, and those who contemplated suicide on the other. But what if someone had problems with both? I understood her perspective, though, because a decade before, and certainly throughout medical school, I would have felt the same way and said the exact same thing.

"Let me take a look at his chart," I told her.

Dr. Davis gave me his name, and I pulled up his medical file on my computer. She had placed three electronic referrals for mental health treatment over the past year. Each time, an administrative clerk called him to schedule; each time, he declined. The primary doctor he'd seen before Dr. Davis had tried to get him to see a psychiatrist too.

There are, of course, many people who don't follow up with medical referrals for all sorts of reasons. But this man kept up with *all* of his appointments with his primary doctor, his pulmonologist, his endocrinologist, and his neurologist. He even attended all of his physical therapy appointments, something patients seemed likelier to disregard. From what I could see, this patient appeared willing to see *any* other doctor. Just not a psychiatrist or anyone else he associated with my specialty.

"So can I tell him to expect your call this afternoon?" Dr. Davis asked me.

I wondered why he'd avoided psychiatrists up until this point. Maybe he was afraid that we'd lock him up on a hospital unit and take away his firearms. Perhaps he thought that we'd poison him with drugs that had irreparable side effects. Or possibly he feared that seeing us would mean that he was "broken" in some way that an actual fractured bone or other physical malady would not.

Within ten minutes, I dialed the man's number. He picked up on the second ring.

"Hello, this is Allen," he said in a raspy voice.

He told me that he was in the parking lot of his granddaughter's school but had a few minutes before her day ended. A few minutes—what could I accomplish in that little time over the telephone with a man I'd never met? Somehow, I had to make a professional judgment of whether he needed psychiatric hospital admission or whether a clinic appointment would suffice, assuming he'd agree to one. These were the sort of stresses I'd dealt with for years while working in psychiatric emergency settings. Just when I thought I had gotten out of that business, Dr. Davis had pulled me back in.

I told him that Dr. Davis was my medical colleague and wanted me to check in as a follow-up to their visit that morning.

"Yes, I really like her," he replied. "She's a good doctor. Very thorough. Just like this."

Without further small talk, I launched straight into the purpose of my call by bringing up the episode with the gun and his granddaughter.

"It's just like I told her," he answered. "I'm fine. I appreciate you calling though."

I sensed he was ready to end the call less than a minute into us talking. I scrambled to keep him on the line until I felt comfortable recommending a plan to Dr. Davis.

"Before this recent incident," I began, "have you ever contemplated or done anything like that before?"

Silence ensued. I thought the call had dropped before he spoke again: "Here and there, you know."

"Was it ever as bad as this last time, or even close to it?"

He paused again. "Well, once, I thought about hanging myself. I made a noose, but I couldn't go through with that."

My back muscles tightened. "How long ago was that?"

"About a week or two after Christmas."

"This past one?" I said as I felt my mouth drying.

"Yes, sir. I let that crazy thinking slip up on me."

It was only mid-March, meaning there had been two episodes of suicide planning and preparation within a three-month period. "This sounds serious," I said. "After your granddaughter is back home and she's with your son, would you be willing to come in to the hospital?"

"I'm okay," he answered. "Like I told Dr. Davis, I feel a lot better. I know it's the devil at work, so I'm going to start back into church. My girl walking in on me was definitely a sign from God."

Just like the psych ER staff had told Dr. Davis, even though Allen was an elevated safety risk given his age and suicide planning, he was not an acute danger to himself or anyone else. Thus, there was no basis to call the police to bring him to the hospital under an involuntary commitment order. My sense was that such a course would only ensure he'd never willingly see a psychiatrist again. I had to call an audible.

"I really think you should come see me. I know Dr. Davis is going to worry about you until someone like me sees you. At least once."

"Okay," Allen said without much hesitation. "I'll do it for her. My wife and I are headed out of town for the weekend to see her parents, but I could come in next week."

My next available appointment was nearly two months out. Way too long to see him. We agreed that he would come the following week in an overbook slot during my lunch break. That wasn't ideal for me, but it was the only option that seemed workable under the circumstances. I called back Dr. Davis and let her know my recommendations.

"Thanks so much," she said. "Thank you. Thank you. I feel so much better now."

"Glad I could help," I said softly, still stressed from the phone call.

"I'm not sure what they're doing to me," Dr. Davis continued, feeling more comfortable now as she launched into a critique of the clinic leadership team. "This morning I saw another guy who'd just gotten out of prison and is staying in a shelter, who only wanted Viagra so he can sleep with prostitutes. It feels like I get all the difficult ones. They keep the more straightforward cases for themselves."

I visualized the nearby detention center and homeless shelter, and the various patients I treated who'd stopped through those destinations. Psychiatrists were a fixture in these worlds, perhaps more than most other medical disciplines. For Dr. Davis and many other doctors, encounters with people on the margins of society like this felt like something too far adrift from what they had envisioned when they started medical school.

As for Allen, despite a clear track record of avoiding psychiatrists and other mental health professionals, maybe this time, perhaps scared by what he'd forced his young granddaughter to witness, he might agree that he needed our help. Or perhaps he'd balk once again, as he'd done so many times before. I'd know in short order.

Soon, I resumed seeing patients back-to-back that afternoon, one thirty-minute visit after another. As the clinic day came to a close, though, my mind flooded with thoughts about the phone calls with Dr. Davis and with Allen. What made so many doctors averse to patients who had mental afflictions, even those much less severe than Allen's situation? And what made these same patients so afraid to see psychiatrists, the doctors presumably best suited to treating them?

On the drive home, I thought about my friends from medical school who were delivering babies, replacing arthritic knees, and removing brain tumors. Or the ones from internship who were interventional cardiologists clearing blocked arteries or oncologists treating breast cancers. As I reflected on my years treating society's castaways in state hospitals, locked wards, and emergency rooms, I wondered if I'd made the right choice.

FOR THE MOST PART, THE GENERAL PUBLIC HOLDS MEDICAL DOC-tors in high regard. We are usually seen as smart, hardworking, committed allies in society's communal fight against the ravages of bodily diseases. The ophthalmologist seeks to restore our vision, the orthopedist our ability to walk and run, the ICU intensivist our life itself. At the center of this physician universe, for the fortunate among us, sits a knowledgeable, personable primary care doctor—the glue that binds together all our medical endeavors.

Psychiatrists, in contrast, are on the margins. More than other disciplines, our work is intangible as we navigate the world of troubled feelings, thoughts, and behaviors rather than concrete physical functions, such as limb movement, blood pressure, urination, or blood glucose metabolism. While most physicians can quantify maladies by seemingly objective data—such as vital signs, heart sounds, imaging studies, or blood tests—the psychiatrist works primarily in the descriptive realm anchored in clinical experience and research. That leads critics of our field, of which there are many, to question our status as a legitimate medical discipline.

Each year for decades, protesters have gathered outside the annual nationwide meeting of the American Psychiatric Association to voice their displeasure with our field. Most opposition these days, however, occurs online and in other media forums. Some claim that we are too cozy with drug companies and have become pill pushers. Others go further, arguing that our diagnoses are not real, our treatments lethal, and that our specialty should not exist. The contrast with other medical disciplines is striking; while physicians of many stripes dispense potentially toxic treatments with uncertain results, there is no dedicated movement to abolish rheumatology or oncology, for example. Antagonism toward psychiatry and psychiatrists at times takes on a political fervor.

Whatever professional disrespect we encounter, the people who seek our care (whose numbers have skyrocketed since the onset of the COVID-19 pandemic) face a far worse reality. Because there is no "lab test" or "lesion" that reliably distinguishes a person suffering a mental disorder from someone who is not (this is true for some "medical" illnesses too), it is easier to discount that person's subjective experience and cast it as something altogether different. The teenager who stays in bed all day is lazy; the woman who cries for hours at a time is weak; the man who consumes too much alcohol or too many drugs is selfish. To make the afflictions worse, these castigations don't just arise from strangers but often those closest to us: parents, siblings, children, and spouses.

I didn't know much about psychiatrists or how hard it might be for people to suffer through serious emotional problems when I entered medical school, other than that I had little interest in either topic. Sure, I'd seen fictionalized versions of psychiatrists treating rich people in posh offices, but that seemed nothing like the doctors on *St. Elsewhere* and *ER*, who were saving people from the brink of death (i.e., "real medicine"). I'd seen homeless people mumbling to themselves in imaginary realities, but mainly, I tried hard to ignore them. When I envisioned becoming a doctor, I saw myself using sutures and stethoscopes; and when I imagined my future patients, I thought about mending injured knees and hearts (literally, not in some mushy, metaphorical way).

Nothing in medical school changed my perceptions of psychiatry and mental illness. In fact, it only solidified them. Many physicians I sought to emulate had little respect for psychiatrists, and some had a seething disdain toward patients diagnosed as mentally ill. This latter sentiment was perhaps best encapsulated for me one day when a well-regarded doctor, after talking to a man with obsessive-compulsive disorder about his options, told his team of residents and students: "Goddamn it, I hate dealing with these psych patients." To him, and many other doctors, interacting with psychiatric patients was a waste of time.

Doctors weren't always the cause of the problem, though. On many occasions, physicians were genuinely concerned about an emotional issue they noticed and would suggest ways a patient might seek help for this distress—only for that person to categorically refuse mental health treatment. Some truly feared they had a serious, undiagnosed medical illness and that focusing on mental health meant the doctor was ignoring their physical ailments. A sizable number, likely carrying the same stigma held by many in the medical profession, went to great lengths to deny that their emotions could have any impact upon their physical health. Nothing could be worse than being deemed "crazy."

My required psychiatry rotation in medical school—the main opportunity to counteract all the negative energy directed against psychiatrists and psychiatric patients—was an epic failure, if the goal was to humanize both sides. The patients I saw on the locked ward were the most severely impaired within this line of work, and the doctors seemed unsettlingly distant and disinterested. At the end of those six isolating weeks, I was eager to return to the bustle of medical life back at the main hospital, imperfect as it was. At least there, we were dealing with patients who usually wanted the help of our medical services. It was a lot easier to wrap your head around the idea of a man experiencing a heart attack than it was a man operating under the delusion that the CIA wanted to assassinate him.

AS MUCH AS WE MIGHT WISH THAT MENTAL HEALTH PROBLEMS, WITH their unsettling behaviors and elusive causes, simply did not exist, millions of people suffer, sometimes to an extreme extent. The National Institute of Mental Health (NIMH) estimates that about 20 percent of US adults live with a mental illness each year. A smaller but sizable number—around 5 percent per year—have what is considered a serious mental illness, one that substantially impairs their lives, whether the cause is schizophrenia or severe forms of depression or bipolar disorder. The impairments range from lost jobs, to broken families, to self-destruction. Suicide is consistently near the top-ten leading causes of death in the US, claiming nearly fifty thousand lives annually in recent years. Over the past two decades, the suicide rate in America increased 30 percent. These afflictions of mental illness occur in men and women, and in the young and old.

There's more. Alcohol, tobacco, and other drugs of potential misuse have been long-standing causes of disability and death. In 2019, the National Institute on Alcohol Abuse and Alcoholism (NIAAA) estimated that nearly fifteen million people met criteria for an alcohol use disorder and that nearly one hundred thousand people die annually from alcohol-related causes. Cigarettes are even worse, contributing to the deaths of over four times that many people each year. And the past decade has brought one media story after another about how opioids—prescribed and otherwise—have damaged families and communities, perhaps overshadowing the larger problem of how they are combined with alcohol, benzodiazepines, and other drugs in all-too-deadly cocktails. In many instances, substance use represents a form of self-medication for underlying emotional distress that goes terribly awry.

Despite the clear burden, it remains difficult for people with mental illness and substance use disorders to receive good health care. Psychiatric hospital beds, limited for all patients, remain largely inaccessible to patients who also have a substance use problem, as inpatient psychiatric facilities are often ill-equipped to treat these disorders and can even deny a patient psychiatric admission on this basis.

Though outpatient treatments are frequently effective, people often struggle to receive care. Some wait months for an appointment, while others can't afford the cost, even with health insurance that seems adequate to cover other medical expenses. The net effect is that too many people wind up in emergency rooms—or in jail—as a last resort. We as a society seem okay with allowing all of this—patients languishing for weeks in emergency departments because of psychiatric hospital bed shortages, people blocked by state politics from lifesaving opioid use disorder treatments, and police required to handcuff people whose major crime is needing transport to a psychiatric hospital. When a system marginalizes mental health, defining it as something alien and less important than physical health, patients pay the price. This is even more true if they are part of a historically marginalized group in America.

Doctors pay too. While many of us in the medical profession would like to distance ourselves from talk of mental illness and substance misuse, the hard truth is that we are some of its biggest victims. Medical students and young residents report higher rates of depression and anxiety than their nonmedical peers, yet for decades, much of medicine persisted in maintaining a punitive culture that discouraged students and practitioners from seeking treatment. Alcohol and drug use is also prevalent. The rate of suicide among physicians exceeds that of the general population. If the stigma associated with psychiatry renders physicians reluctant to seek care themselves, it's no surprise that this attitude translates to the care that they provide to their patients. The marginalization of mental illness within medicine is bad for patients, and it's bad for doctors too.

SO WHY DID I END UP CHOOSING MEDICAL LIFE AS A PSYCHIATRIST, placing myself on the margins of medicine in a field I once loathed? It wasn't a lack of options—at the time, I was comfortably enrolled in a well-regarded general medical residency program where I would be able later to specialize in cardiology or to work as a primary care sports medicine doctor. Further, with a prestigious law degree, I had many opportunities outside of medicine. Looking back, there wasn't a singular event that set me on this path but rather a series of encounters—most with patients, but also crucial ones with family, friends, and colleagues—that awakened me to the ubiquitous nature of mental health distress and the yawning chasm between what people needed and what they received. I believe I could have become a good cardiologist or team physician, but psychiatry is where I felt I could make the biggest impact.

While mental health problems and the field of psychiatry remain marginalized, the extended isolation and changing social norms imposed by the COVID-19 pandemic brought heightened attention to these areas for a larger swath of the population. Rates of anxiety and depression disorders increased across virtually all demographic groups; alcohol and other drug use even more so. Intimate partner violence rates rose. The public gained increased appreciation for the psychological trauma black, Asian, and other marginalized groups face. There is a lot of psychic suffering to go around.

As we've resumed our lives in the post-COVID world, we've been presented with the chance to redouble our attention toward addressing the burden of mental illness. For starters, we need to change how we educate future doctors and other health care providers about psychiatry and behavioral health. A few weeks working on a hospital psychiatric unit simply won't do. On a policy level, we have enforced a separation of medical and behavioral services, which results in poor access to mental health care and compromised medical outcomes. We have made inadequately trained law enforcement officers—much to their dismay—the default option when people face emotional crises. The all-too-frequent criminalization of mental health– and drug-related problems speaks volumes about our society's fear, ignorance, and apathy toward those who suffer from them. The pages that follow will take you through my experiences as a medical student, intern, and psychiatrist as I incorporate stories of patients and doctors who have faced these struggles head-on and are seeking change.

The need is urgent. Every day across the country, people with underlying behavioral and emotional problems arrive in America's clinics and hospitals. Too many of them leave having received no treatment for this distress or, at best, substandard care. Until that reality is no longer true, patients and doctors will continue to ail. We have the opportunity within medicine, law, and health policy to break through these layers of marginalization, instead of merely reinforcing and reflecting society's long-standing bias toward mental illness.

PART I

FAILING DOCTORS

1

MISEDUCATION

THE OMINOUS SIGNS BEGAN TO APPEAR AS SOON AS I LEFT THE highway. Turn left for the federal prison. Right for the juvenile detention center. Straight ahead for the alcohol and drug treatment facility. I had taken a detour from the traditional hospital and clinic settings I was used to and entered a hidden world where society puts those it doesn't want to think about. What happened to the institutionalized people out here, and what was going to happen to me? Instinctively, I double-checked to be sure my car doors were locked.

On this cold, foggy winter morning in rural North Carolina, I was about to start the first day of my six-week psychiatry clerkship. Till then, my clinical experiences in medical school at Duke had taken place in mainstream hospitals and outpatient clinics, where I'd worked alongside surgeons, general internists, and family physicians. For my psychiatry rotation, however, I'd been assigned to a state-run psychiatric hospital, a place devoted exclusively to the treatment of mentally ill people. Knowing nothing about such hospitals when I'd started the clinical year of medical school a few months earlier, I had been partially reassured by vague comments from more senior students, throwaway lines like "You'll learn a lot there."

In the week leading up to my start date, however, current classmates who had rotated at the hospital started issuing not-so-cryptic warnings:

Don't turn your back on a patient. Don't stay in a room by yourself with one either. Don't allow a patient to sit between you and the door. Don't wear a necktie lest it get used to choke you. They made the place sound like a jail or prison, at least the kind I'd seen on television and in movies. I figured they were exaggerating, or that if they were genuinely afraid, my experience as an oversize black man would be radically different. Until I saw the road signs. By then, it was too late to change course.

By that point in the academic year, I'd logged four months in clinical settings: two on the surgical service at our main hospital and another two at a family practice clinic in a medical park near campus. The state hospital, in contrast, was twenty miles away, in a different county. The location itself hadn't seemed odd to me until I saw what other institutions were nearby. Suddenly, it felt as if I had crossed some kind of invisible boundary. Was psychiatry going to be as distant from other medical fields as the state hospital was from the other clinical locations I'd known? Was this the best way to teach medical students about treating mental illness?

My heart fluttered as I approached the parking lot. This place didn't look like the hospitals I'd seen in and around Duke, nor like the half dozen or so I'd visited during my medical school interviews a few years earlier. Instead of a multistory design that housed emergency wings, surgical suites, and medical beds, this hospital was a vast expanse of old, interconnected, single-floor brick buildings. It resembled a barracks. Or a jail. As I left the car, I noticed my knuckles aching from having gripped the steering wheel so tightly.

Nothing about the building I entered brought to mind a medical setting. I saw no doctors or nurses, no front desk check-in window where staff asked for health insurance cards, no patients seated in a waiting area, no signs for laboratory or X-ray. Instead, it felt like I'd walked into a rural, county government office. Quiet. Sedentary. Overlooked. Moments later, I joined three classmates in a midsize administrative conference room for an orientation session.

A muscular, middle-aged man with thick, graying hair and suntanned skin introduced himself to us as a security supervisor. *Why aren't we meeting with a doctor, nurse, or other medical staff? Is this really a hospital?* I thought.

"Is this everyone?" he asked.

We looked around and nodded collectively.

"Good. No girls this time around. It's always easier when it's that way."

That sounded nearly identical to what I'd heard from an older surgeon months earlier. Both felt men were physically and emotionally better suited to "difficult work" and seemed to long for the bygone era when medical students were overwhelmingly male. His words were unquestionably sexist, yet in the moment, when my focus was inward and not on what his attitude might mean for my female classmates, I let his comments pass by without much thought. Maybe working at a psychiatric hospital, despite initial impressions, wasn't going to be so different from the months I'd spent in operating rooms and surgery wards.

A half hour later, after we had completed administrative paperwork, we received the temporary ID badges and keys that would enable us to circulate around the hospital. I clipped the badge to my shirt and placed the keys on the ring next to those for my apartment and my car.

"Make sure you look around before you open the door on a unit," the man told us. "Patients have been known to try to elope. That's bad for everybody."

On that upbeat note, he escorted us to the building that housed the patients. Moments later, each of us went our separate ways and met the pair of staff members we'd be working alongside for the next six weeks. Given his diatribe about women and safety, I was surprised to see that my supervisor was a woman, just as I had been the one week when I worked under the direction of a female surgeon. This psychiatrist had short brunette hair and a light olive complexion. She appeared fortyish. DR. BEAL was printed in black block letters on her ID badge.

"Hello," she said to me softly before quickly turning her gaze toward her colleague.

"I'm Alice," said the shorter, younger woman who stood next to Dr. Beal. "I'm the social worker working with Dr. Beal."

Before medical school, I'd only thought of social workers as the people who got involved with child protection cases or to help people receive government assistance. During my rotations in surgery and family medicine, however, I'd learned how important they were in making things happen in the medical sphere: getting patients transferred from one hospital to another hospital or to a different medical facility; coordinating the array of outpatient medical services some need after being discharged from the hospital; and so on. At this hospital, each psychiatrist paired with a social worker, who did similar tasks.

I followed Dr. Beal and Alice down a long hallway as they carefully opened the door and entered a male-only patient ward. In contrast to the medical and surgical floors at Duke and other general hospitals, these units were separated by gender. The goal was to prevent consensual or unwanted physical interaction (at least of the heterosexual variety), which reinforced my impression of the place as a correctional facility. Dr. Beal seemed to sense my unease.

"Have you been inside a psychiatric unit before?" she asked me.

I told her I'd seen emergency departments, operating rooms, medical floors, and intensive care units, but never a psych ward. "It's very different from a regular hospital," I said.

"You'll get used to it after a few days," she assured me.

My anxiety ebbed a few notches as we walked toward the central nursing station and the first few patients breezed right past without noticing me. While I had seamlessly blended in with my surroundings a few years earlier on the basketball court as a college athlete, the opposite had proved true in hospitals or clinics, and in most other areas of life. Day in and day out during my medical school rotations, as a six-foot-six black male, I'd get some combination of "How tall are you?" or "Wow, you're tall," or "Do you play basketball?" or "Where do you play?" or "Can I have your autograph?"

Yet here on this unit, the patients seemingly had more pressing things on their minds than whether I had a good jump shot or could dunk with both hands.

"Can you let me out of here?" asked a man approaching me with desperate eyes. "I don't belong in here with all these crazy people."

He had a smallish frame, leathery skin, and patchy, gray facial hair. Obviously, he didn't agree with his doctors about being in the hospital. I looked over to Alice and Dr. Beal, who both ignored his pleas. They told me he was assigned to a different medical team. I followed their lead and started to walk past him. He shifted tactics.

"If you can't do that, can you at least get me my smoking privileges?"

Why would a hospital give patients smoking privileges? I wondered.

Seconds later, another patient approached, his eyes wide, hair matted, and teeth yellowed. The smell of his breath caused me to hold mine while he spoke.

"I need to use the phone to call the police," he asserted, his voice filled with conviction. "I need to reach DPD. I'm being falsely imprisoned by the CIA and FBI. I think ABC, CBS, and NBC will want to know about this. CNN too."

My head hurt trying to process the barrage of three-letter acronyms and how they might connect to the man uttering them.

"Welcome to our world," Dr. Beal said, smiling for one of the few times I saw during that rotation. "Wearing the white coat makes you stick out like a sore thumb on the unit."

I'd remembered to ditch my necktie, a staple on other rotations. Apparently, the white coat was optional too. Dr. Beal wore a tan blazer as her top layer; Alice, a powder-blue blouse. Classmates on the pediatric service rarely wore their white coats, as they'd been told that garb might frighten some of the younger children. I wondered if my white coat was having the same effect on some psychiatric patients. Maybe the people who I thought had ignored me had avoided me out of fear. As I looked at Dr. Beal and Alice, then glanced down at my white coat, I realized that sexism wasn't the only reason a patient might see the three of us and reasonably conclude that I was the "medical" person.

Toward the end of the rectangular hallway, we approached Gene, a young man who paced in a fashion that mimicked the geometric dimensions of the unit.

"Good morning," Dr. Beal said to him. "How are you today?"

He stared at us—me, as the new face, longer than the others—then looked away.

"I'm fine," he mumbled.

The unit housed adults eighteen years old and above, which made Gene the thinnest walking and talking adult I had ever seen. He was probably six two (his mini-Afro made him seem even taller) but could not have weighed more than 120 pounds. The hospital-issued pants that barely fit his waist stopped mid-calf, and his torso seemed completely lost inside his top. Aside from scraggly hair around his chin and mouth, and a few creases across his forehead suggesting some wear and tear in his life, he could have been a gangly prepubescent sixth grader on his way to becoming seven feet tall.

"Is there anything you'd like to discuss with us in private?" Dr. Beal asked.

He shook his head. During my surgery rotation, patients had their own hospital rooms where we spoke with them daily as they recuperated, as did patients at the family medicine clinic. Here, though, we were more likely to chat with patients—at least those who had been there a few days—in full view and earshot of others. Neither doctor nor patient seemed to mind it much; in fact, it seemed preferred by both parties. It was the exact opposite of the psychiatry stereotype, where a person lies on the therapist's couch in a secluded office. Maybe it was as simple—and problematic—as the difference between what a wealthier, private-pay person could receive compared with what a poorer, largely black, group of patients could get. Or maybe, in this correctional-like setting, both doctor and patient were wary of the other, so they mutually agreed to keep interactions, whenever possible, in plain sight of others.

"How did you do with breakfast?" Dr. Beal asked Gene. "One of the goals we talked about yesterday was for you to try to eat each meal."

"I only want apples," he replied as he scanned the area around us and then glanced toward the floor. "Apple a day keeps the doctor away. But you all keep bothering me."

Dr. Beal and Alice suppressed smiles. It would have been funny if we had been in an ordinary setting talking with a healthy person.

"It looks like you refused the medication that we ordered for you," Dr. Beal said.

"I only need apples," he replied.

"Okay," Dr. Beal said. "We'll see you tomorrow."

That was it? This thirty-second exchange seemed to accomplish nothing based on what I'd seen from doctors elsewhere. Dr. Beal didn't ask any of the usual medical questions about pain, bodily functions, and the like that I'd heard recited to one patient after another. Even more surprising, she didn't probe his mind much either with questions about his mood, anxiety levels, or sleep patterns. But we did know that he wasn't eating his food as Dr. Beal wanted and that he refused whatever drug she had prescribed. Perhaps, for her purposes, those were all the details that mattered.

"He's really skinny," I said as we walked down the hallway toward the central nursing station. "Does he have an eating disorder?"

"He has schizophrenia," Dr. Beal told me. "This is his second time here. Part of his delusion is that he is being poisoned, although for some reason, he's latched on to apples as a safe food. He thinks his parents are trying to kill him to collect on a life insurance policy."

Alice then explained to me that no such policy existed. She said that people such as Gene were unlikely to qualify for good life insurance anyway.

"Why?" I asked.

"Because people with schizophrenia die about ten or fifteen years sooner than the average person," she answered. "For insurance companies, that puts him at high risk."

I tried to envision how terrifying it must have been to be convinced that your parents were poisoning you and, from the other side, to be a parent unable to reach your son lost in the clutches of psychosis. But these emotions reached me only at some surface level. I couldn't imagine anyone I knew thinking or acting in this way. He reminded me of the dozens of downtrodden homeless men I had seen over the years, people I could keep safely at a distance up until then. Though I was standing in a hospital ward, a place where someone in his mental state could improve, I couldn't connect with his plight in the way I could a woman whose appendix was removed and now felt better. Anyone could get appendicitis. But not schizophrenia, I told myself.

"Is he at risk of serious health problems," I asked, "from being so skinny?"

"Not in the short term," Dr. Beal answered. "All his tests were essentially normal. Long term, it could definitely be a problem. The medication I ordered should get rid of those delusions. Plus it has the added benefit of weight gain as a side effect."

"But I thought he refused to take it?"

"He'll get it today," she replied in a matter-of-fact tone.

I looked at her, genuinely confused. He didn't seem like he was easily persuadable.

"It's different here than it is on your other rotations," she said.

Dr. Beal explained the hospital's policy on forced medication. One of her psychiatrist colleagues had seen Gene that morning and agreed with her assessment that this approach was needed for him to improve. Starting later that day, each time he refused to take his prescribed pill, he would be forced to receive an injectable form of an antipsychotic drug in his rear end. Eventually, she told me, he would take the pill form when a nurse offered it to him. Eventually.

My jaw slacked. On my surgery rotation, our team had a patient who refused insulin to treat his diabetes. After a few contentious days, they agreed to discharge him home against medical advice once he had sufficiently recuperated from his operation. Despite the serious health risks, no one talked about forcing him to receive insulin. The consensus, as I understood it then, was that people had the right to make poor decisions, even if this caused serious disability or even death. All we could do was present them with the facts and hope they reconsidered.

But Dr. Beal explained that patients with schizophrenia lacked the understanding to know that they were sick in the first place, and thus the guideposts for approaching their situation differed. I didn't know what to make of that distinction. All I knew was I couldn't imagine being the doctor to ever give such an order.

As Dr. Beal moved on to seeing other patients on our list, I thought about everything I'd seen and heard that morning. I had entered another reality, one where few rules or procedures I'd been taught so far in medical school seemed to apply. Learning about forced medication policies felt about as useful to practicing surgery or family medicine as powerlifting was for a concert violinist.

My miseducation in psychiatry had begun.

FOR LUNCH THAT DAY, JIM, A PSYCHIATRY RESIDENT A FEW YEARS removed from medical school, took my three classmates and me to a local sub shop. As we waited for our food, one of us mentioned the proximity of the psychiatric hospital to prisons and various behavioral treatment facilities, as I'd observed that morning.

"Not so good for the property values," Jim said.

We smiled. This trio of classmates all came from families where home ownership was a given. One had a radiologist father. Another had a pediatrician mom. The third had parents who worked as university professors. I'd also grown up in a house my parents owned, though their jobs hadn't required college degrees. In contrast, I suspected—and confirmed later—that many of the patients and custodial staff at the hospital came from worlds where *property values* was not part of the regular vernacular.

"This town feels like the setting for one of those horror movies," another classmate said. "You know, with the prisoners and the psych patients escaping into the streets."

"Definitely," the third one responded as I nodded in agreement.

Jim started to speak, then paused, as if considering censoring himself, before finally deciding against it. "Some of us have been saying for a long time," he began as a smile came across his face, "that if someone were to nuke this town, the social problems of central North Carolina

would just go away. We'd just have to make sure they gave all of us notice to get out of town before it detonated."

One classmate laughed out loud, almost spilling his drink. The rest
of us looked at each other awkwardly, unsure how to react. We then
responded in uncomfortable ways—muffled groans, hands over face,
headshaking—that people often do after hearing off-color jokes. As a
resident, Jim was our most immediate mentor and supervisor, and none
of us wanted to start off a new rotation telling him that what he'd said
was cruel.

On my surgery rotation, I had heard some doctors say harsh things
about overweight patients, or those with poor hygiene, or people who
challenged them in ways that upset them. But I thought psychiatrists
were supposed to be "nice" doctors, the ones trained to deal with some
of society's most challenging people, seeing the best in them as they
tried to help them. Instead, Jim was suggesting that the world would be
better off if a certain swath of institutionalized people, and the places
designed to help them, simply didn't exist. Clearly, he assumed that
neither we nor anyone we cared about had ever experienced, or could
ever experience, a severe mental health problem requiring a stint at that
state hospital.

What I didn't know then, and what Jim didn't seem to know either,
was that psychiatrists had played an important role in the tragic,
immoral eugenics movements that peaked in late nineteenth- and early
twentieth-century Europe and America. If he had, I'd like to think
he wouldn't have made that joke, and that if I'd known this sordid
history, I might have found the courage to push back against him. I
hoped so, anyway.

When I returned to the hospital after lunch, Dr. Beal told me that
she had meetings that afternoon and asked me to check in with Alice,
our social worker. Alice welcomed me into her cramped office. She told
me that she'd just spoken with the mother of Gene—our super-skinny
patient with schizophrenia—to update her on his status.

"I told her that Dr. Beal was going to start him on a new medication today," she said, "and that we hoped he was well enough in a few days for her to come see him."

"Did you tell her about the forced medication process?" I asked.

"Not in detail. But she wants us to do anything we can to make him better."

I tried to imagine the desperation Gene's mom felt. My parents would have been heartbroken to see me in that way. "How do visiting hours work here?" I asked.

Alice explained that a patient had to be behaviorally stable enough to sit in an office for a family meeting to occur. "To be honest, we don't get visitors that much for most of the patients," she said. "I think for a lot of families, it's too much. He's lucky in that regard."

I thought back to my time on the surgical units, where I saw patients in the intensive care unit after bypass surgery or major abdominal operations. Not only was it easier for me to imagine having a heart attack or colon cancer than being psychotic or suicidal, but seeing these people flanked by wives, husbands, and children anchored them to a human world outside of tubes, IV lines, and monitors. Without visitors, the patients at the state hospital too often lacked that connection to a life outside the hospital, and I could see how that disconnect might make it easier for doctors to keep their distance too.

Toward the end of that day, as I finished looking through the chart of the last patient on our assigned team, I heard a disturbance in the area outside the nursing station. Jim was talking to a patient. I couldn't make out what Jim said to him, but the patient's words were loud and clear.

"You made a mistake," he said in a threatening voice. "Now you're going to feel what it's like to have no control when I put my fist down your throat and you stop breathing."

"Sir, you can't talk like that to anyone here on the unit," one of the nurses responded.

"Screw you, bitch," the patient sneered back at her.

Jim looked over to this nurse. "Give him five of Haldol."

Haloperidol, or Haldol, is a powerful drug used to treat psychosis, especially to tamp down agitation and aggression, as it can be given by injection. I had moved from where I'd been seated to a spot where I could observe Jim's interaction with the patient, staring at it like it was the scene of a bad car accident. The man looked to be midthirties. He was unshaven and overweight. A large vein bulged in his neck. His face was flushed.

For some reason, perhaps because of my size or because I was new to the unit, his rabid eyes met mine. "Why are you looking at me like that? Are you a sissy or something?"

I wanted to run back to the staff work area, grab my backpack, and get the hell away from this hospital. But my feet were glued to the floor. Within a few seconds, four large men in their twenties and thirties came into view and surrounded this patient at a distance. The seemingly oldest one in the group told the patient that the nurse needed to give him some medication and that it would be a lot easier on everyone if he calmed down and allowed her to do her job. Just then, the same nurse that this patient had cursed calmly approached him with a syringe filled with liquid medicine.

"I'm not taking that shit," the patient snarled.

Suddenly, the four men converged on the patient and took him down to the floor like a quarterback sacked on an all-out blitz. Two men held his legs while the other two secured his arms. The nurse pulled down his pants and injected the tranquilizing medication into his butt.

The patient growled, "You're all going to hell. And I'm going to come find you there and eat your intestines."

So this was what Dr. Beal meant when she said that Gene was going to take the medication she prescribed, whether he agreed to it or not. Shocked, I stumbled back toward the workstation area. One of the ward assistants approached me.

"Having fun yet?" he asked.

Not at all, I thought. I longed to scrub in and watch a backbreaking, six-hour cardiac bypass operation. Or to be so busy at the family medicine clinic seeing one patient after another that I missed lunch. I didn't know then how unusual this day was for most psychiatrists in practice, as few routinely order forced medication or see patients who physically threaten them. Nor was I aware that most mental health care treatment that people receive doesn't even involve a psychiatrist. All I knew about psychiatry on day one was that I wanted absolutely no part of it.

AT EVERY US MEDICAL SCHOOL, PSYCHIATRY IS A REQUIRED ROTA-tion alongside foundational fields, such as pediatrics, general hospital medicine, surgery, and obstetrics. In most cases, students spend that entire time working on a psychiatric unit, just as I did during my rotation at the state hospital. While an important part of doctoring in any field is being able to distinguish between acute illness requiring emergency medical care, and everything else, the hospital-only approach to psychiatry education has clear drawbacks. Especially when 95 percent of medical students will become something other than psychiatrists.

At the hospital where I was introduced to psychiatry, the majority of the patients were diagnosed with schizophrenia, bipolar I disorder (the severest form), or a related condition along that spectrum. As important as it is for psychiatrists, first responders, and the social safety net to better address the needs of this all-too-neglected and vulnerable group, most mental health problems that an average nonpsychiatrist doctor sees fall far outside these categories.

Major depression is about twenty times more common than schizophrenia. Anxiety disorders, which include panic disorder, generalized anxiety disorder, and others, are nearly ten times more prevalent than bipolar disorder. Those are the mental health conditions afflicting people that the average doctor encounters most often. Yet at the state hospital, patients with primary depression or anxiety came to our attention only after they had tried to kill themselves, or when their impairments caused them to stop eating and drinking, or they posed some serious threat to a spouse or child. Not once during medical school did I see the inside of an outpatient psychiatric clinic, the kind of setting where more than 90 percent of people who visit psychiatrists receive their care. This disconnect would be like students learning about family medicine practice without ever working in a primary care clinic, or a surgery rotation where students didn't work in an operating room.

"It was nothing like I thought it would be," Dr. Jeff Drayer told me. "I came to medical school thinking I might become a psychiatrist. And then I did the rotation."

Drayer—a dermatologist and accomplished television writer—arrived at Duke two years before I had and did his psychiatry rotation at the nearby veterans' hospital. Like me, all he essentially saw was a tense psychiatric unit.

"Everyone seemed to be in such terrible shape," he said. "And the only solution seemed to be to give them drugs that had terrible side effects."

By focusing so singularly on psychiatric hospitals—and those serving the most seriously ill at that—the traditional psychiatry rotation for medical students potentially warps their view of what psychiatrists do and who psychiatric patients are. Some who might choose the profession are dissuaded by the false impression that most psychiatric patients are tortured and dysfunctional, which in turn creates a view of psychiatrists as nothing more than caretakers of people with poor life prospects.

Dr. Diana McNeill, a diabetes specialist and widely recognized leader in medical education, offered similar commentary about her own psychiatry experience at Duke nearly two decades earlier.

"I remember going to the top floor where the psychiatry patients were admitted and thinking that these people were so isolated," she told me. "It didn't seem therapeutic at all."

The experiences Drayer and McNeill highlighted were by no means limited to Duke. Doctors who attended state medical schools in New Jersey, Missouri, and Utah have told me similar stories, as have those who went to private schools, such as Harvard and Yale. The many rewards of working in psychiatry, such as helping people through bereavement, divorce, and other life challenges, or reducing disabling depression and anxiety symptoms so that a person can return to work or school, were too often rendered invisible in the crucible of locked wards.

"I needed to see some patients who were doing well managing their mental illness," Dr. McNeill said to me as she described her psychiatric rotation in med school. "If all one sees are patients with uncontrolled, complicated diabetes, one thinks that is how all patients are with diabetes; the same can be said about patients with mental health issues."

This dissatisfaction with the rotation permeated my classmates' experiences. During the second week of my rotation, I was back on campus at Duke for a weekly series of lectures, which brought together all students currently on the psychiatry rotation. During a midmorning break, several of us went downstairs to the cafeteria for coffee and bagels. We began comparing notes on our respective experiences. A classmate described working with a psychiatrist who admitted patients from the emergency department, but never conducted a physical exam where he touched a patient. Not once.

"I think that's how they all are," said Pete, an aspiring cancer specialist. "It probably has to do with that whole boundary thing you hear about where they think patients will take it the wrong way."

He was talking about the stereotyped perception of a psychiatrist romancing an emotionally vulnerable patient. During a medical ethics session a few months earlier, our lecturer had talked about the need for us to guard against inappropriate relationships with patients. He mentioned that this could occur in any medical field, but made a point of singling out psychiatry and gynecology.

"Or maybe they just aren't any good at hands-on doctor stuff?" said Anne, who was interested in pediatrics. "And that's why they chose psychiatry."

A few of us nodded in agreement, oblivious to how arrogant we sounded in suggesting that certain medical school graduates were inferior to others—or that, as second-year medical students, we might know more about medicine than people who had completed four years of medical school and then gone on to spend additional time as interns and residents in various medical settings.

"I don't think psychiatrists should even go to medical school," Pete said finally. "There should be a separate type of school where they can learn about psych meds and street drugs. Maybe it could be combined with graduate school psychology programs."

This led us to question why we were required to do the psychiatry rotation in the first place, rather than use those six weeks in the emergency department or on another medical or surgical service. Only one student pushed back on our collective psychiatry bashing.

"But what about the cases where a person has a medical problem that presents with psychiatric symptoms, or the opposite?" asked Betty, who was interested in primary care and was spending her weeks with a team of psychiatrists who took consults from the medicine and surgery services. "Doesn't the psychiatrist need medical training for that?"

The rest of us stared at each other in silence. What she said made sense, but it didn't sound like anything we had actually seen during our rotations. Some students were on psychiatry units completely separated from the rest of the general hospital. Four of us were at a state facility, miles away from the nearest regular hospital. If the intent of our curriculum was to show that psychiatry belonged on equal footing with other medical disciplines, with all of them working together for the patients' benefit, then the medical teaching program had failed. Conversely, if the goal was to marginalize psychiatry from the rest of medicine, and to show how different psychiatric patients were from medical or surgical patients, then the system was getting exactly the results it was designed to achieve.

BY THE END OF OUR PSYCHIATRY ROTATION, WE'D LEARNED THE clinical diagnostic criteria for schizophrenia, mood disorders, and various anxiety disorders. We knew the different types of medications used to treat these conditions, proposed theories on how they worked, and the potential side effects that required monitoring. We'd also been taught that there were people who had personality disorders that interfered with their ability to get along with everyone around them. And people who dealt with severe alcohol and drug problems. Neither of these latter groups responded much to psychiatric medications: psychotherapy was the preferred approach, only we didn't get to see that in action. Still, we comfortably passed the national exams for psychiatry training. We'd checked the medical education box.

Perhaps this would have been fine if everyone with emotional and psychological issues was confined to psychiatric hospitals or specialized psych wards and emergency rooms. Or for those stabler patients, psychiatric offices tucked away from the rest of the health care system. But the reality is that anywhere a doctor is regularly seeing conscious patients, there is a good chance mental health issues will eventually be involved.

According to a 2014 report, a review of medical records showed that approximately 20 percent of primary care office visits involved managing mental health–related diagnoses. When the context was expanded to include substance use problems and the emotional factors involved with diet, physical activity, and pain, the percentage of encounters involving behavioral health concerns likely exceeded half of all visits. There is no reason to believe that these numbers have declined in the past decade. If anything, the COVID-19 pandemic, increased political polarization, and escalating social isolation have increased demand for mental health services that far outstrips supply.

While depression, anxiety, and substance misuse—frequently the result of psychological or physical trauma—are the usual suspects that intrude into people's lives and into doctor-patient encounters, the typical medical student remains inadequately exposed to these topics. And once they graduate and begin work in nonpsychiatric fields, formal instruction on mental health is minimal or nonexistent, leaving their earlier medical student psychiatry clerkships as the only formal training that they ever received. As a result, day after day, patients bring to their primary care providers and other medical specialists every form of overlapping mental and physical distress, and these doctors too often don't recognize the mental health issues or don't know how to begin treating them.

After finishing my psychiatry rotation at the state hospital and returning to the main medical campus for subsequent rotations, I witnessed how this marginalization of mental health problems hurt patients. I especially noted it on the general medicine service, where I spent the final eight weeks of my clinical year. Many of the patients had heart disease, and of that group, most had a major risk factor—cigarette smoking—which was technically classified as a psychiatric disorder (nicotine dependence or tobacco use disorder) in textbooks and on billing forms. Yet as the weeks went on, I observed that almost no medical professionals treated it that way.

As students, we were taught to multiply the daily number of smoked cigarettes by the number of years smoked (pack-years) to assess heart disease and lung cancer risks. After those numbers were entered into the patient's chart, however, pretty much nothing happened. Some doctors did prescribe nicotine replacement patches or gum. But during my time in medical school, others were concerned these drugs might worsen heart disease, at least in the short term while patients were in the hospital. I couldn't recall at that point hearing anyone discuss the psychological dimensions of why patients smoked, what might be triggering their behavior, or what might motivate them to quit. I brought this up to my supervising medical resident one evening while admitting a sixty-five-year-old man with heart failure, who had smoked since he was fifteen years old.

"You can't really do anything for it," the resident said, raising his hands in the classic gesture of surrender. "They have to do it all for themselves."

Was it really that simple? That some people were "strong" and could quit smoking, and others were "weak" and couldn't—and thus did not deserve our extra effort? Or had our medical education failed us? Through repeated exposure, we learned the lesson that a doctor's job extended only to "fixing" conditions that responded to medication or surgery. Every other kind of problem, whether it was smoking, alcohol use, or obesity, no matter how much it complicated the health of patients, was not the doctor's problem. And for years, I didn't have the time or perspective to ask, "Then whose problem is it?"

Toward the end of that general medicine rotation, a man I had been monitoring got transferred to the cardiac intensive care unit after his initial blood test indicated he'd suffered a heart attack. Following a cardiac catheterization procedure, he returned to our service to recover further before being discharged home. As I skimmed through his chart, I noted that the cardiac ICU doctor had recommended sertraline, an antidepressant drug, and, more interestingly, devoted several lines about counseling the patient on quitting smoking and eating a better diet. I was intrigued and asked the resident about this doctor.

"He thinks treating depression is as important as controlling blood pressure or lowering cholesterol," the resident responded with clear skepticism. "He gave a lunch talk to all of us a few months ago about his theories. He's also big on all that mind-body stuff. Yoga, Pilates, and meditation."

At the time, with my limited view of the world, I regarded yoga and meditation as something that rich white women did in fancy gyms and offices. I hadn't even heard of Pilates. But the premise—that active efforts to achieve a better mental state could improve physical health—seemed perfectly logical to me. How, then, had I gone through nearly an entire year of hospital training without hearing anything of that sort, from either the psychiatrists or other physicians I'd encountered, until I came across one hospital note from a single doctor?

This doctor's perspective connected with me not just professionally but personally. My blood pressure had been consistently elevated for more than a year, and as I researched how I might treat it, I felt apprehensive about taking medication for the rest of my life. Some research professors at Duke and elsewhere were investigating the effectiveness of nondrug options—exercise, diet, and stress management—to address heart disease and its many risk factors. Eventually, I decided to contact one of them, and after a thirty-minute conversation in which he gave me an overview of his current work, I agreed to spend my third year of medical school working in his clinical laboratory.

There, during my time away from the hospital, I began to understand various aspects of the mind-body interface. Hundreds of scientific articles had been written on the ways that psychological stress worsened physical health, and I became fascinated learning how different nondrug interventions generated measurable improvements in study participants.

Yet little of this data seemed to translate to what I'd seen in clinical practice. Often, the patients we saw were too sick to apply these techniques in a meaningful way, at least in the short-term setting in which we treated them. But just as important, the health education system left us too tired, too busy, and too unknowledgeable about preventive and mind-body interventions to help patients beyond the realm of drugs and procedures.

When I returned to the hospital for my fourth and final year of medical school, I decided to spend the required subinternship—the most rigorous four weeks of that year—in Duke's cardiac intensive care unit. There, it was life and death for the patients in the most literal sense, and functioning as close to an intern—a brand-new doctor—as a medical student could, I was present to see much of it, day and night. Both physically and emotionally, the experience was simultaneously exhilarating and exhausting.

About midway through the rotation, I arrived at the unit on a Monday morning after a much-needed day off. Among the dozen or so patients for us to see, one stood out. Michelle was not the sickest, nor the youngest, nor even necessarily the most tragic. In room after room, each patient battled different forms of life-threatening heart disease—blocked arteries, heart failure, and irregular rhythms. But Michelle was the only one whose own immediate action had landed her there. The day before, she had taken an overdose of an antidepressant medication with the intention of killing herself. The drug had significantly altered the electric circuitry in her heart, prompting her admission to the cardiac ICU.

At this point, I hadn't given psychiatry or psychiatric patients much thought in the nearly two years since my second-year psychiatry rotation had ended. As we approached Michelle's room, the cardiology trainees and medicine residents assigned to the unit seemed to be practicing a similar kind of avoidance. Until now, they'd been socially engaged with each patient, asking one man about his years as a race car driver, the woman next door to him about her travels to Asia, and so on. Near Michelle's room, however, everything changed. The doctors spent more time outside the room discussing her case than they had with the other patients, and that talk focused exclusively on her cardiac monitor readouts and lab results. Her suicide attempt, the reason she had been hospitalized, wasn't mentioned.

"Do we need to go in?" one of the medical residents asked hesitantly.

The cardiology fellow—the most senior person in the group at that moment—peeked into the room, where Michelle was sleeping.

"She seems fine," he said. "Her heart rhythm looks good. Let's not disturb her. We don't want to overwhelm her with too many people right now."

We then moved on to the next room, where the doctors regained their friendly demeanor. I wondered what made them see Michelle as so different compared with the rest of the patients. Perhaps they feared saying or doing something that would make things worse. Or maybe they were afraid that if we spent too much time with her or looked too deeply into her soul, then whatever afflicted her might transfer onto us. Whatever the reason, these doctors seemed to be avoiding emotional connection with Michelle in much the same way that some psychiatrists had eschewed physical contact with their patients.

A short while later, Dr. Lewis, the cardiologist on duty to supervise the unit that week, arrived. Boyishly slender, he looked like the type of doctor who never took the elevator, limited his carb intake, and played tennis several hours each week. Annoyingly energetic.

"Are we ready to get started?" he asked.

The cardiology fellow and the medical residents reviewed the list of patients as we stood outside each room. When we got to Michelle's room, one of the medical residents began explaining her case. After the resident had reviewed all of the important heart-related concerns, Dr. Lewis started his inquiry.

"Do you know why she was prescribed this medication?"

Michelle was taking a drug belonging to a class known as *tricyclic antidepressants*. Doctors prescribed them to treat things other than depression, such as chronic headaches. The resident assumed it was for depression, given that the patient had taken an overdose.

"Do we know if she is getting it from her primary care doc or a psychiatrist?"

The resident looked stumped again. He shook his head.

Dr. Lewis kept on: "If it's for depression, doesn't seem like she should have been on it, given its risk in overdose. That is one of many reasons we prefer the newer SSRI drugs, which are a lot safer."

The resident looked over to his supervising cardiology fellow, who came to his aid: "We figured we'd just page Psych and let them figure all that out," he said.

Dr. Lewis sighed. The cardiology fellow and resident looked away, embarrassed.

Only after this exchange finished did it all come together. Dr. Lewis was the cardiologist whose note I had read as a second-year medical student, the one my supervising resident at the time derisively said was interested in "all that mind-body stuff." Later that morning, I found myself standing next to Dr. Lewis in the break room as he was pouring himself a cup of tea.

"How is your subintern experience treating you?" he asked me.

"I'm enjoying it," I said honestly.

Then I switched gears. "You seem to know a lot about psychiatry," I said. "More than a lot of the other doctors I've worked with before."

He smiled. "I initially thought I might go into the field," he said. "My uncle was a psychiatrist, and he seemed to enjoy his work. But my psychiatry rotation in med school was at a county hospital ward, and during my first week there, this scary guy punched a nurse and knocked out some of her teeth. I decided right then to cross it off my list."

"My psych rotation wasn't much better," I said.

Over the ensuing years, I had heard many doctors say similar things—that they'd initially been interested in psychiatry until they rotated onto a psychiatry ward that seemed like a prison and appeared to require psychiatrists to be wardens.

"But it's still important to be knowledgeable about the basics of mental health and the latest developments," Dr. Lewis continued. "I feel like no matter what field you go into, this stuff will keep coming up with your patients."

After Dr. Lewis left, I continued thinking about my psychiatry experiences. While the state hospital had helped me gain an appreciation for the gravity of severe mental illness, the whole concept still felt distant, like misfortunes that happened to "other" people, not anyone I cared about or would ever know. It would take a much more personal encounter with mental distress for me to begin connecting with psychiatry on a deeper level.

2

DISSONANCE

I STOOD IN A REAR CORNER OF THE EMERGENCY DEPARTMENT, MY feet pasted to the floor, staring at the patient my senior resident had sent me to interview. He stared back, frowning. My heart jumped in my chest. *I knew this guy!* Scott and I had played pickup basketball together many times—at least twice a month during my early days in medical school, when he was a college student. It had been more than three years since I'd seen him.

He didn't seem to recognize me, which caused my stomach to sink. I was now a medical intern, and the stress of hospital life had taken its toll: my hairline had begun receding, and I'd lost fifteen pounds since we'd last seen each other. Had I aged that much in the interim, or did I look that much different in a white coat and loafers from how I did in a T-shirt and high-tops? This was my first time encountering someone as a patient whom I'd known outside the hospital. But Scott wasn't in the locations where broken legs, appendicitis, or bloody diarrhea were evaluated. Instead, we were in the psychiatric area. What the hell was he doing there?

Altered mental status (AMS). My supervisor said that's what had brought Scott to the hospital. A nonspecific phrase to describe a sudden or gradual change in brain function, it's a term we use in medicine as often and easily as we use words like *fever, cough, headache,* or *pain.* All sorts of medical problems can cause AMS—ranging from abnormal blood sugar levels, to drug intoxication, to an assortment of brain infections. But based on what my resident had told me about Scott, the doctors who'd seen him so far didn't think any of those problems were at work. Instead, their gut told them that he was a "psych case."

Our role as general medicine providers was to monitor him and assess for these medical problems, to clear him for psychiatric admission. I'd been part of this process before, but suddenly, it made no sense. Because now they were talking about *Scott*, someone I'd known as a good student, fit athlete, and friendly and social guy. How could a psychiatric illness—serious enough to cause altered mental status—be describing the person I'd shared so many hours with on the basketball court? How could Scott be this restless, wide-eyed person who didn't even recognize me now?

STIGMA AND MALICE TOWARD THOSE WITH MENTAL ILLNESS HAVE taken many forms throughout history without ever going away. The religious persecutions of the Middle Ages became the vicious asylums of the seventeenth and eighteenth centuries. The twentieth century gave us eugenics and lobotomies, among other shameful practices. And while it's easy, and perhaps comforting, to point out the especially bad actors in history—doctors and hospitals motivated by pride and greed—the reality is that many of us still look down on those with mental illness. This stigma takes different forms and is commonly expressed in one of the following three responses: denial, moral judgment, and fear/avoidance. I had experienced all of these reactions within my own family during my formative years, nearly two decades before I found myself in the ER with Scott.

In some of my earliest memories, I'm sitting in my maternal grandmother's one-bedroom inner-city apartment on Sunday mornings, watching her pace back and forth, cigarette in hand, as she talks with my mom about her various concerns. I was about nine or ten years old when Grandma mentioned to my mom that a friend had suggested that she was "too high-strung" and that this might be bad for her blood pressure.

"This is who I am," Grandma said defiantly, her finger pointing into the air as if answering back to that friend in live time. "There is no other way for me to be."

She argued with her invisible opponent, standing from her seat as if delivering a dramatic closing argument. Anyone would be "high-strung," she asserted, if they'd had a life like hers: Growing up poor in a family of twelve kids in the Jim Crow South. Having a daughter die at eighteen months. Working as a maid and raising three kids as a single mom after her husband abandoned them. The fact that she constantly expected bad things to happen, and that she needed to stay one step ahead of them was, in her view, exercising essential survival skills for a difficult life. This led to harsh judgments of others who seemed, in her eyes, to lack those tools. Her other daughter, my aunt, was "high-strung" too—pacing, smoking, worrying, anticipating the worst from situations—but also prone to crying spells and periods of reclusive behavior. Grandma had no patience for that, only condemnation.

"She's letting herself go," Grandma said to my mom, with anger in her voice. "She's giving up."

Their exchange became too much for my child brain to process; as they talked back and forth, I went into her kitchen and helped myself to a stack of cookies.

"Your grandmother and aunt have too many things going on for me," my mom said to me a few hours later on the drive home.

My mom had long seen herself as the stable one in her family: married, with two children who did well in school and steered clear of trouble. She felt that she could control only her own life and couldn't invest too much time and energy trying to help her mom or sister with their emotional troubles. Any further discussion of family mental health issues, as I can recall, was tabled for many years.

I didn't know it then, but I suspect both Grandma and my aunt suffered—to different degrees—under the weight of trying to live up to the Strong Black Woman archetype, which stresses the value of independence, resilience, and control in the face of an unkind outside world. Black people in their universe, and women in particular, didn't have time to dwell on their feelings. Certainly not outside the home, in any case: there was too much to be done to keep their lives afloat. My mom embraced this ethos too, only more successfully, and she surely passed some elements of it down to me.

When I was growing up, I also saw the fear and avoidance that so often characterizes public stigma toward those with mental illness. Where I lived, there were folks that you knew to steer clear of. One particular woman in our neighborhood stood out. She was generally pleasant on calm days, but was prone to episodes of emotional outbursts directed toward her children that would spill out of her household into view of those of us nearby. The general consensus on our street was that her neighbors wanted her to move away, but while she remained there, everyone should keep a safe distance from her. "Something is wrong with her," people said, but what that was, or what that might mean for her life and those of the people around her, I never heard discussed. I accepted what I'd seen and been told: it was better not to get involved.

Because I didn't recognize them as stigma, these attitudes remained with me as I got older and informed my interactions with people who likely had different types of psychiatric issues. In high school, a girl that had scratched up her wrists because she got a B-plus on a test "needed to get a grip"; in college, it was much easier to be part of a group that joked about a socially awkward guy than spend a half hour talking with him one-on-one. And, of course, the homeless men and women I'd drive past day after day, disheveled and delusional, these were people you simply avoided. Although I had entered medical school without any real preformed opinions about treating pneumonia or colon cancer, I'd arrived with a preconceived bias against mentally ill people. One that I was unaware of.

On the day my troubled patient turned out to be a former friend, and where I was forced to face these personal shortcomings, none of these issues had been at the top of my mind. Long term, I was interested in a career that seemed to have little in common with psychiatry; short term, I was just desperate to take a nap.

IT WAS A RAINY SATURDAY MORNING A FEW MONTHS INTO MY GEN-
eral medicine internship, the first year I worked in a hospital with the
letters *M.D.* after my name. Life on the general medicine floor meant
taking care of people with bread-and-butter health problems: heart disease, pneumonia, and intestinal bleeding, with a few exotic illnesses
thrown into the mix. For many of us, the three-year medicine residency
training program served as the required stepping stone to future spe-
cialization. Cardiology was my top choice: each month, it seemed, a new
drug or device propelled us forward in battling against the most common cause of death.

At that moment, however, I was at the midway point of a twelve-day
stretch without a day off and simply wanted to get through my thirty-
hour shift without too much damage to me or anyone under my care. I
sat in a physician workroom, finishing up a daily progress note on one
of my patients.

Trey, a senior third-year resident who was headed off in a few months
to a cardiology program in New York, was filling in for the second-year
medical resident I'd been working with that month. That resident had
called out sick with a bad case of vomiting he'd gotten from food poisoning. I'd expected Trey to be furious about being brought in on such
short notice to work on a Saturday, but he seemed calm.

"They're paying extra for the time," he'd told me when we'd chatted
a few hours earlier. "Good money. I've got crazy loans to pay, so it's cool.
Plus, he's solid, so I won't be cleaning up a lot of crap. And I've heard
you're solid too."

With Trey in the driver's seat, we breezed through morning rounds
for our list of patients in about half the time it normally took during
the weekday. Since our patients were all stable, Trey was eager to
watch a pregame show for that Saturday's slate of college football
games, while I hoped to lie down for as long as I could. Just a few
months into internship, I'd embraced its mantra: "Eat, sleep, and pee
whenever you can."

I'd completed most of my patient notes and was eagerly anticipating
a power nap when Trey's pager activated. My positive energy abruptly

dissolved and quickly refashioned itself as indigestion as I awaited his report. After a few minutes of back-and-forth with an emergency department doctor, Trey hung up the phone and shook his head.

"Sounds like we got a psycho one," he said.

Throughout medical school, I'd heard doctors use terms like *psycho*, *crazy*, or *nutty* to describe patients many times. Some part of me knew this was wrong, the same way it was to speak in demeaning terms about morbidly obese people. But compared with the racist, sexist, and homophobic things I'd heard, it barely registered in my mind. I assumed they'd probably had unsettling experiences like my psychiatry rotation at the state hospital.

"What do you mean?" I asked Trey as I felt my stomach flutter with nervous dread.

"Our new admit is a twenty-four-year-old man who is manic—probably bipolar, they say—who was brought in after he got into a scuffle late last night with some homeless dudes outside a McDonald's."

"Injuries?" I asked, my brain running through possibilities for why he would be coming to our medical service rather than an orthopedic or neurological service.

"Nothing serious. He's got some cuts and scrapes. Head CT scan was normal. Ortho is going to take a closer look at his hand X-ray. Might have a subtle fracture."

"Drugs?" I asked.

"His urine was clean. No alcohol in his system either."

I felt my neck and shoulder muscles tightening. "Why are they calling us?" I asked. "Sounds like a slam-dunk psych case."

"Well," Trey began as a smile came across his face. "This isn't your average patient. Mom and Dad are lawyers, and it sounds like they want the executive workup done. And nobody around here wants to make these lawyers upset."

During a medical school lecture on professionalism, a professor told us that the patients and families that we had to be most careful around, aside from other doctors and nurses, were journalists (who could bring unwanted attention to us) and lawyers (who could sue us). It sounded like the doctors in the emergency department treating this patient had received a similar warning.

"Are there certain special lab tests they want done?" I asked.

"The whole enchilada. But we can only do so much on the weekend."

"Damn," I replied, squelching the other four-letter words that came to mind.

I shouldn't have been so upset. We were one of the admitting medical teams that day, so we were going to get patients added to our list. Better they come to us earlier in the day so we could reach our "cap"—the top allowable number of new patients in a day—sooner, so as to increase our chances of sleep during the night. Yet that logic failed to calm me. The continuous eighty-hour weeks were already beating me down, with each new admission feeling like a calamitous burden. Many times, I'd heard older doctors say that these working conditions would make us better doctors in the end. But I was increasingly losing faith in those assurances.

"All is not lost," Trey said. "Basically, you just have to babysit him over the weekend. Worst case, the Med-Psych team will take him on Monday. They're good docs."

The Med-Psych team was led by doctors trained in both general medicine and psychiatry. They didn't admit patients over the weekend but typically picked up a few that came in on Saturday or Sunday. The week before, I had transferred an elderly man with schizophrenia and a bad foot infection to their team.

"And think about how much worse of a case you could have gotten than someone who is basically healthy and most likely just needs to get back on his lithium or whatever the hot new 'bipolar' drug is these days," Trey continued.

I calmed down a bit as I took in his words. Trey was cynical, for sure, but practical and efficient—two traits welcomed on any hospital ward. Downstairs, I followed the winding hallway to the emergency department, where my hospital badge activated an electronic device from red to green, which opened the double set of wooden doors. Instantly, the flurry of action heightened my senses. Doctors, nurses, nurse aides, and radiology techs moved with purpose as if at a busy city subway station, where each patient room represented a stop on the route.

As I joined the throng, it suddenly dawned on me that despite many trips to the emergency department as a medical student and intern to admit patients, I'd never been to the psychiatric wing. Based on my memories of the state hospital, that suited me fine.

"Can I help you?" a woman asked as she turned toward me, her voice partially muffled by the thick window that separated us.

The psychiatry wing was situated in the rear corner of the emergency department, essentially cordoned off from the areas where doctors took care of emergency-sounding problems like strokes and car accident injuries. Through a plexiglass window adjacent to a wooden door, I saw two hospital staff, a man and a woman, looking at monitors showing multiple views of people dressed in hospital pajamas. My badge didn't allow me access to this room.

"I'm from Medicine. They called us about an admission," I said, referring to the name Trey had given me.

"Well, he's actually in that room right down there," she answered, pointing to the hallway behind me. "Come in and I'll tell you more."

Her badge indicated she was a nurse. Midfifties, with graying hair pulled back in a ponytail, Margaret opened the door and introduced herself. The twentysomething man with her was a nursing assistant. I quickly took in my surroundings. This workroom was about the size of an average medical clinic exam space and had the customary digital blood pressure machine and sharps container for used needles that one finds in medical clinics of all types.

But that's where the similarities ended. Straight ahead through another plexiglass window (this type a one-way mirror) and another locked door, I saw an open area divided into six small cubicles, each consisting of a lounge chair bolted to the floor and a small television secured on the adjacent wall. In one cubicle, an older man vacantly watched a game show, while in another space, a small woman paced in circles. A third patient sat on the floor with her knees crossed as she scratched her armpits. Watching these people through one-way glass felt like viewing

them at a police station or county jail. A large monitor in the nurses' station showed live surveillance images similar to those from a big-chain
grocery or department store.

"First time here, huh?" Margaret asked, smiling.

"That obvious?" I responded.

"It definitely takes some getting used to."

I noticed that the monitor showed images of two rooms—currently
empty—with padded walls, bare except for what looked like a rectangular concrete slab at one corner.

"Are those your seclusion rooms?" I asked.

Margaret nodded. "As for your guy," she began, "well, he's sick enough
to be back here with our other patients."

By "sick," she meant the extent of his psychological impairment. I'd
learned during medical school that psychiatric patients were described
that way when they were either psychotic or manic to such a degree that
normal communication bordered on the impossible. The term was also
applied to people whose suicide risk was extreme.

"But with his parents," she continued, "the doctors decided it would
be better for him to be in one of those rooms just outside. We typically
use them for people who aren't as sick or if they have medical problems
that might be too much for us to handle back here."

I felt myself becoming irritated by the preferential treatment this
patient and his family were receiving. Reflexively, my mind filled with
stereotyped assumptions: that the patient was white, that his parents belonged to a country club, drove luxury cars, and had traveled extensively.
Those were the sort of people I'd seen get special rooms in hospitals, have
chef-catered meals prepared for them, and who were able to get medical
students or interns removed from their care. Only here, in the psychiatric
area, this seemed far more radical and unfair, as it meant the difference
between having your own room versus being placed behind two locked
doors in what seemed, from my vantage point, like an alphabet soup of
mental illness. My narrow-minded thinking wanted this patient to have
it just like the others, rather than considering why everyone else didn't
get better accommodations in the first place.

Margaret told her assistant that she would be right back as she led me out of the locked area and into the main hallway. Less than twenty feet from the psychiatric unit, she stopped outside at the first door on our left. She stepped into the room.

"Hello," she said to my new patient, as she glanced back at my ID badge and gestured for me to follow her inside. "This is Dr. Tweedy. He's one of the doctors who will be taking care of you upstairs."

My body froze as our eyes met. The young man was black. Sadly, despite having met at least a few thousand professionally educated black people by this point of my life, I still defaulted to the assumption that someone with two parents who were lawyers was white. But his brown skin was just prelude to a much larger shock.

I heard the patient say something and Margaret reply but couldn't make out their words. It felt like I was in a bad dream. When my feet were finally able to move, they backpedaled me into the hallway. Margaret followed.

"We'll be right back," she said to him, before turning to me. "Are you okay?"

"I know him," I whispered.

Her eyes widened. She waited for me to say more.

"I mean, I haven't seen him in a while. It's been years, actually, but . . ."

"You never expected to see him here," she answered, completing my thought for me.

I wondered if I should even be his doctor. Teachers had discouraged us at different times throughout our medical training from treating family and friends, because our judgment in those situations could be compromised. But Scott and I didn't have a real relationship. I hadn't seen or spoken to him in three years, maybe longer. I'd never even known his last name, which is why I had no reaction when I saw Scott's full name on his electronic medical chart.

"He's super bright," I said. "When I knew him back when he was in college, he talked about going to law school and then getting into politics."

I went on about how smart, athletic, and ambitious Scott had been in those days, as if that might inoculate him from psychological problems.

During my weeks at the state hospital, the patients were severely ill—so much so that regular, everyday conversation with them was often not feasible. Of course, they deserved to be treated with respect, but since I knew them only in their states of mental sickness, I viewed them as fundamentally different from patients I saw on other rotations. As I understood it then, these were folks who'd had something terrible happen to them, something we didn't really understand, and the best we could do was to keep them calm so they didn't hurt themselves, or, more important, harm someone else. It was as if, on some semiconscious level, the usual goals and responsibilities of medicine—to partner with people in distress to ease their suffering and improve their lives—did not fully apply to this group of patients.

Margaret listened patiently to my glowing descriptions of Scott before stating something I'd never really considered:

"That's the thing about mental illness," she said. "It's an equal-opportunity bitch."

I stood silently for a few seconds as I absorbed her words. Then my pager activated. Someone upstairs needed a higher dose of pain medicine. This request brought me back to the moment. I was a busy intern. I needed to get started with my admission paperwork for Scott before someone else arrived or one of the elderly folks on our team started to crash. I didn't have time to dwell on the ubiquity or unfairness of mental illness.

"Thanks for your help," I told Margaret. "I'll go see him and check in with you after."

"You sure?" she asked. "Maybe it isn't such a good idea."

Backing out would have meant Trey or someone else needing to complete the admission for Scott. As interns, one of the things we feared most was being seen as weak. Being a young doctor required mental toughness. Fulfilling one's responsibilities.

"I'll be fine," I said. "But thanks for listening to me."

Margaret reluctantly went back to her secured area while I stepped toward Scott's room. I tapped on the full-length sliding glass window.

"Come in," he said.

Scott sat on the edge of the bed, his butt resting uncomfortably on the mattress as if he had hemorrhoids. His feet, covered with hospital-issue socks, tapped the floor in a rhythmic pattern. He wore an oversize hospital gown that opened in the back. His right hand was scraped up along his knuckles, and his left forearm had several horizontal scratch marks. His lower lip had been bleeding recently, and his left eye appeared to be in the early stage of swelling. It looked like he'd been in a minor car accident. Or gone a few tough rounds in a street fight.

As we made eye contact, Scott stared back without an ounce of recognition, waiting for me to speak. The intensity of his glare unnerved me. Normally, I would have started things by giving a typical doctor spiel, introducing myself and asking him what sequence of events brought him to the hospital. But I wanted to see if I could stir his memory first.

"We knew each other a few years ago," I began. "Do you remember me?"

He frowned. "From where?"

"I'm Damon," I said. "We used to play basketball together. Back when you were in college. You know, pickup games in the afternoons. Lots of them."

Scott scanned my face for a few seconds, then down at my feet before our eyes locked again. Confusion slowly gave way to excitement. "Oh yeah. Damon. Lefty jumper."

I felt a wave of calm caress me. His mentioning that I was left-handed meant that he wasn't simply pretending to remember me. Maybe he hadn't lost his mind after all. Maybe this was all just a short-term problem that would resolve itself quickly.

"I didn't recognize you in the white coat," he said.

I smiled. He'd known me only in basketball gear. He seemed to be thinking logically.

A woman's cough shook me from my reminiscing. We weren't alone. "Would you like me to step out?" she asked through her thick African accent.

The woman sat in a chair next to Scott's bed. A pop-diet book—one promising a thirty-pound weight loss in thirty days—rested in her lap.

Her role was to function as a sitter, someone to keep eyes on a patient at all times and alert staff if that person started to act erratically. Her presence was a jarring reminder of our situation. I'd grown accustomed to sitters for elderly patients with dementia. But Scott did not fit that description. Not at all. Instead, he had been deemed "crazy."

"Sure," I said to her.

Scott and I were now alone. I stepped closer to him. We exchanged a man hug—a handshake followed by a quick one-armed embrace. But then I immediately questioned if I should have done that—I was the doctor and he was the patient.

"So you're a grown-up doctor," he said. "In your fancy whites."

I smiled uncomfortably. I started to ask Scott what he'd been doing since college. Then I thought about Trey describing him as "bipolar" and the nurse labeling him "sick," and worried I might not want to know the answer. The note from the psychiatry resident, which I assumed contained those details, hadn't been completed. My data was scant.

"Other than the cuts and scrapes I'm seeing, how are you feeling right now?" I asked.

He yawned. As I looked more closely, I noticed that his eyes were bloodshot. But if he was feeling tired, he fought the exhaustion. Without warning, he slid his body onto the bed, reclined, and did a set of abdominal crunches. Then he sat up and shadowboxed—left, right, left—for a set of ten. Finally, he went through a repetition of alternating leg lifts. The whole thing took about a minute. "That feels better," he said.

Attempting to think like a psychiatrist might, I tried to interpret his sudden burst of energy. Was this a sign of troubling hyperactivity?

"How did you find out I was here?" he asked.

"Coincidence," I said. "I happen to be on a medical team that's been assigned to admit you today."

Scott looked confused. "Like I told those other doctors, I don't think I needed to come in to the hospital. Nothing's seriously broken, and they said my head scan checked out fine. But I appreciate all the care you guys have provided."

I wondered if he understood that I wasn't an orthopedic surgeon, neurologist, or emergency medicine doctor involved with evaluating his injuries. Or that the doctors who'd seen him so far thought he had a serious psychiatric problem. Unsure how to ask that, I focused on his visible injuries. "Looks like you got into a pretty serious fight," I said.

"Yeah, man. I was waiting for a call at this pay phone, and this homeless-looking dude wouldn't get off the phone. I told him that I had to take a call from the governor."

"The governor?" I asked as my stomach began to flutter. "What governor?"

"The one from our state, man. I was just getting ready to file my papers."

I had a bad feeling about where this conversation was headed, but I couldn't stop.

"What do you mean?"

"I'm running for the Senate."

I frowned. "The state senate?"

He shook his head dismissively. "That's peanuts, man. I'm talking the US Senate."

I broke eye contact and quickly looked around the room, up and down, side to side, to regain my bearings. This was not a weird dream. We were indeed in the emergency area of the hospital. And a person I'd known years before was talking utter nonsense.

"But you're too young for the age requirement," I said. "You aren't thirty yet."

"I'm going to get a special waiver," he said, his eyes widened. "I wrote a letter to the governor. That's what the call was about. He was going to grant me an exemption."

I detached for a moment and tried to recall the symptom checklist for a manic state I'd memorized in medical school. This sounded like a grandiose delusion, like my quitting my hospital job with the plan that an NBA franchise would give me a roster spot, even though I was, on my very best days, merely an average college player.

I knew that bipolar disorder wasn't the only cause of mania. My brain searched for scenarios I'd learned about over the years. Even though his alcohol and drug screen results had come back with no signs of either, could he have ingested something they didn't test for? There was also the possibility of him having had a bad reaction to a prescription medication or having some rare unidentified medical problem that came with psychiatric symptoms. When he was just some abstract patient, I had bristled at the idea of his parents demanding we chase down obscure diagnoses—what we called *medical zebras*. But now that this patient was *Scott*, I wanted to do the same.

"So are you with the surgeons?" Scott asked, the pace and tone of his words becoming more urgent. "One of them was supposed to take a closer look at my hand."

"I'm with the medicine team. The surgeons and psychiatrists are separate—"

He cut me off midsentence. "What? Are you one of those damn shrinks too?!"

"No, no," I protested, as if he'd accused me of trying to steal his girlfriend or his identity. "I'm definitely not a psychiatrist. I'm with the general medicine team. We deal with things like the heart and lungs, liver and kidneys, blood infections, and stuff like that. I have to do this part of my training to get where I want, which is to be a heart specialist."

Scott didn't seem to hear my response, as he continued to fume about psychiatrists.

"Why do they waste your time in medical school with that crap?" he said. "Those guys aren't real doctors. I was just starting to feel better the past few months and now they want to start drugging me up again. That's all they do."

I felt my neck clench. Scott had apparently had previous encounters with psychiatrists, making me worry that his mental concerns might be more chronic.

"Can you get me out of here?" he asked. "I've got so much to do. You know, at first I was mad about missing the governor's call. But now I'm thinking that I can spin all this in a way to help my campaign. It will make me seem more human to the voters."

I clearly understood why the emergency department doctors didn't feel comfortable sending him home. And also why the orthopedic surgeons, if his hand was indeed broken, wouldn't want to cast it until he started thinking more logically.

"I think you need to make sure everything is well with you before you worry about getting out of here," I said.

He glared at me. "You sound like those other doctors. You know, I'm starting to wonder if my hand is injured at all or if this is some kind of bullshit way to keep me in the hospital so they can drug me up again. It doesn't really hurt that bad."

I felt myself losing control of the interview. This is where as a medical student I would have turned to a physician to take over, but a few months into my internship, I was still adjusting to the reality that *I'm the doctor*. I wanted to call Trey. If Scott had been crashing in some medical way— dangerously high or low vital signs, a life-threatening heart rhythm, his liver or kidneys failing—it would have been a no-brainer. That is what he'd been trained to treat. But Trey couldn't help with Scott's illogical thinking any more than I could.

"Can you get me out of here or not?" Scott persisted.

I assumed the other doctors who'd seen him already explained this to him. He was considered a "voluntary" admission, as he'd come in by ambulance after his altercation, but I imagined that if he physically tried to leave, the psychiatrists would get involved and convert his status to "involuntary." Maybe they'd had this conversation with him, but in his current mental state, he didn't understand, or perhaps my arrival had given him hope that I could rescue him and expedite his discharge. I sighed.

"I don't think that's possible right now until all of the doctors clear you to go home."

Scott closed his eyes and clenched his fists for a second. Then he scanned the room, as if looking for a hidden camera. "Are you a plant?"

"What . . . what do you mean?"

"Did they send you in here to get secret information on me, knowing that I would let my guard down?"

The psychiatric checklist from medical school came to mind again. This is what was called a *paranoid delusion*.

"Scott, you're not making any sense," I pleaded with him. "It's just like I said from the beginning. I'm on the medical team. I had no idea that I would be seeing you until the emergency department called us."

He turned his head away from me. "Get the hell out of my room."

"But, Scott—"

"Get the hell out of my room now!" he yelled as he turned back to me and stared with fire in his eyes. "If you don't leave now, I'm going to call the police. I also want a lawyer. It's my constitutional right. I don't have to answer any more of your questions."

I stumbled backward, twisting my ankle slightly. My trembling hands struggled to open the sliding glass door. Finally, I escaped the room, my heart pounding, my own mind struggling to connect to reality. *What the hell had happened to Scott?*

IN MEDICAL SCHOOL, AS WE LEARNED ABOUT THE VAST ARRAY OF things that can go awry with the human body, a handful of diseases stood out to us for reasons of self-interest. Over 90 percent of us were in our twenties, and so our attention heightened when the professors described diseases that people were more likely to develop as twenty- and thirty-somethings, in contrast to most others, which had a predilection for the aged. Acute leukemias and lymphomas were the scariest, but autoimmune and inflammatory disorders—multiple sclerosis, lupus, Crohn's disease, to name a few—were more common and pretty harrowing in their own right. Young men could get testicular cancer, while young women might develop endometriosis. Our amplified responses to hearing about these illnesses has its own term, *medical student syndrome*, to suggest that medical students and other young health care trainees are prone to develop health-related anxiety during their studies.

Schizophrenia and bipolar disorder follow a similar trajectory, often announcing themselves to those in their twenties; in fact, it is quite uncommon for someone to be diagnosed with either condition in middle-age or beyond. But I don't recall learning about these disorders during the classroom-based lectures or hearing classmates discuss them then; or maybe I blocked out my professor's words because I never seriously considered that either condition could happen to me or someone in my life.

The first time I remember talking with classmates about how psychiatric illness often targeted young adults occurred the next year during my rotation at the state hospital. The four of us assigned there worked with doctors who kept different caseloads and schedules, but at least once each week we tried to meet up for lunch. On one such day, Carson described a patient who compulsively drank so much water that he'd nearly killed himself months earlier.

"Man, it would really suck to be schizophrenic," John said.

"It's worse than cancer," Carson responded. "Even if you get stage IV lung or pancreatic cancer, there's a chance you'll beat it. And if you don't, you'll be put out of your misery soon enough. This feels like infinite torture."

"Yeah, it's really gotta suck for the parents," Teddy chimed in.

I agreed with everything they'd said. While physical illnesses could disrupt and damage lives in myriad ways, mental illness, at least what we saw at the state hospital, seemed to strip people of their identities and transform them into something less than human. With physical ailments, we'd seen as medical students that there were gradations of disease: some people with diabetes had terrible complications while others were essentially healthy. Sure, some people could lead normal lives with anxiety, depression, and alcohol-related problems. But bipolar disorder or schizophrenia? No chance, based on what we'd seen and heard. We didn't know about exceptional people like Elyn Saks or Kay Redfield Jamison, prolific intellectuals despite having schizophrenia and severe bipolar illness, respectively. Nor did we know about the everyday person with either illness who nonetheless maintained a functional life.

Instead, when someone arrived at the state hospital with what the psychiatrists described as "first break" or "first episode" symptoms, an air of gloom filled our workspace. We could see their future all around us, in the patients who'd been hospitalized time and again. These images circulated through my mind as I found myself confronted with a

manic, paranoid version of the Scott I'd once known. I prayed that his
fate would be less grim.

I WENT BACK TO THE MAIN PSYCHIATRY AREA AFTER MY STUNNED
retreat from Scott's room. Margaret, the nurse, opened the initial locked
door and let me inside the small workroom. Her assistant had gone through
the second locked door into the area where the patients were housed,
and appeared to be helping the older man with using the restroom. In
her assistant's place, a short, bearded guy with light-brownish hair and
freckles stood next to Margaret. I could tell from his ID badge that he
was the psychiatry resident on duty. He was heading to see one of the
patients in the locked area, but stopped as I entered. I introduced myself
as part of the general medicine team.

"So you're here to admit our young guy for his executive physical?"
he asked me. "Nice to have friends—or in his case, parents—in high
places, right?"

I stared back at him. I didn't like his sarcasm. But I couldn't get too
judgmental, considering I'd felt the same way when I thought the patient was some anonymous rich kid. Everything changed for me when
I saw it was Scott.

"I suppose," I said. "But I wouldn't want to be in his shoes right now."

I glanced at Margaret, whose face looked pained. From her reaction,
and the resident's callousness, I could tell that she hadn't shared my con-
fession of knowing Scott.

"You're right," the resident conceded as he glanced through the plexiglass window into the locked area. "No one like us would want to be
on the other side if we could help it. Guess I can't blame his parents for
keeping him out of here."

He spoke to me as a fellow doctor. Similarly, Scott was well-educated,
and, the last time I'd seen him years before, was on the path to becoming a lawyer like his parents. In my naive, classist, self-deluded view of
the world, the resident's "like us" category made sense: we weren't the
kind of individuals who were supposed to end up sharing close quarters

with homeless people, criminally prone people, drug-addicted people, all of whom I'd come across over the years in ample supply at the state hospital and in various emergency rooms.

"Got any questions for me?" the psych resident asked.

"Yes," I said hesitantly. "Is there any chance that, you know, the way he is acting is caused by drugs or a bad reaction to something?"

He shook his head slowly. "I really don't think so. His urine and blood tests were clean. And he was adamant about not taking any drugs, including over-the-counter supplements. He went on and on about how the voters are looking up to him and that he has to set a good example for the children to impress their parents."

That sounded exactly like the delusional way Scott had talked to me. If external culprits couldn't explain his distorted thinking, then I desperately wanted it to be something internal that could be identified on a lab test and definitively treated.

"What about a medical condition, you know, like a thyroid problem?" I asked.

"Doubtful. His physical exam is pretty benign, and so are his basic blood tests, so I don't suspect any kind of metabolic problem going on that would cause this. His CT scan was normal too. But I guess that's up to you guys upstairs to search for zebras. To be honest, if this were your average person off the street, the people we usually see here, we would have already sent him to the psych floor. No questions asked."

I thought back to my psychiatry rotation in medical school. Many of those patients started in emergency departments before they were transported to our facility. From what I recalled, those transfer notes were pretty bare. While they usually had urine drug screen results and data on blood pressure, temperature, and heart rate, the reports often came without blood tests or any indication that the patient had received a real physical exam. Because the state hospital accepted those without health insurance or with Medicaid, while many other psych hospitals did not, our population skewed poor. And disproportionately black. For the first time, I wondered how many of those people might have been undertreated and potentially misdiagnosed.

"So you're thinking this is all psych-related?" I asked.

He nodded. "This looks like textbook mania from bipolar disorder. He's previously been diagnosed with depression. Sometimes it takes a while for the manic part to develop."

My heart sank. "What do you recommend as far as psych meds?" I asked.

He suggested the combination of haloperidol, a powerful antipsychotic medicine, and lorazepam, a sedative, while we were doing our additional medical workup. Once it was settled that his issues were psychiatric, he recommended that we switch to lithium, a classic treatment for bipolar disorder, and risperidone, then a newer antipsychotic medication.

"I'm almost done with my note," he said as he glanced back through the one-way mirror, where the woman who had been scratching her armpits was now trying to get another patient to do this for her. "Once we get her situated," he said, referring to the woman, "I'll finish it up."

"Thanks," I said, averting my gaze from her, desperate to free myself from this alternate universe. I could try to recall Scott as the smart, vital person I'd known. But the other patients, strangers to me, I just didn't know what to think of them. And that made me uneasy.

After the psychiatry resident entered the patient area, Margaret turned to me and spoke: "I figured it wasn't my place to tell him that this was your friend from the past."

"Thanks," I said.

We talked for a few minutes, Margaret assuring me that Scott would be treated in a dignified way. She then shared something from her life that put everything into context.

"I know what this is like," she said, "only in a much more personal way. My sister was diagnosed with bipolar disorder when I was in high school. She was hospitalized for a month after she tried to kill herself. It sent our family down a path we never imagined."

Perhaps the greatest cruelty of severe mental illness is that it so often announces itself when people are in their late teens or early- to midtwenties. Ordinarily, at least in our collective imagination, these years are the time when one's life is full of vigor and opportunity. Family and friends share in that optimism. But for Margaret, her parents, and Scott's parents, this same phase of life for their loved one brought confusion, anguish, displacement, and dread of an uncertain future.

AFTER LEAVING THE EMERGENCY DEPARTMENT AND HEADING UPSTAIRS to the medicine floor, I quickly became consumed with medical intern life again. The man in room 813, a retired high school principal who'd told me stories about the challenges of school desegregation in the 1970s, reported chest pain, so I had to order an EKG and blood tests to check whether he was having a heart attack. The woman in room 821, a retired nurse who showed signs of early-stage dementia, spiked a fever and required the standard workup of a chest X-ray along with blood and urine tests. A young man in room 827 with gastrointestinal bleeding needed a blood transfusion.

In the midst of managing one mini-crisis after another, Scott's situation got pushed to the back of my mind. This medical work—physically examining people, monitoring their vital signs, lab tests, X-ray results, and EKG tracings, and making clinical decisions based on them—as stressful as it could be, still felt much more comfortable than talking to a manic, delusional person. The "data" that came with these general medicine duties imparted a sense of control that our decisions were grounded in facts, however limited, ambiguous, or conflicting those might become at times.

But what if schizophrenia and manic depression were indeed similarly biochemical illnesses, as some psychiatrists had told us in medical school during our second-year rotation, only not nearly as well understood because of the immense complexity of the brain? Could that mean that rather than being "less medical" as we typically regarded psychiatrists and the mental disorders they treated, these severe illnesses, on a scientific level, were perhaps "more medical" given their underlying intricacies? Would that reduce the stigma? Maybe, but I wasn't so sure. Scott's illness exhibited behavioral changes that had physically unnerved me in a way that a person hospitalized with an aggressive form of leukemia simply did not.

Around midafternoon, I sat down to write Scott's admission note and saw on the computer screen that he'd been brought from the emergency department to our floor. Trey, the senior resident working with me that day, entered the physician workroom a few minutes later. We'd last talked that morning before I went to see Scott.

"I just checked in on our psych guy," he said to me. "He's sleeping from the Haldol and Ativan they gave him downstairs in the ED. Nothing else going on with him right now."

I thought about mentioning that the "psych guy" was someone I'd known from my past. But a part of me felt embarrassed—for Scott certainly—but also for myself, for reasons I didn't understand. I kept quiet.

"Actually, there is one thing," Trey continued. "Our guy's mom has been ringing the operator number off the hook. I think the psych people down in the ED should have talked to her, but I guess at this point, he's ours."

"What should I tell her?" I asked, feeling helpless.

"I mean she needs to understand that he's come in on the weekend, so right now we are focused on life-and-death medical stuff. We can check his thyroid and parathyroid levels. But basically, nothing else is going to happen test-wise until Monday."

Thyroid and parathyroid are small glands in the neck area that control metabolism, temperature regulation, calcium levels, and many other bodily functions. Psychiatric disturbances can occur when their hormone secretions are aberrant.

"Should we order an MRI?"

Trey threw up his hands. "With his normal head CT, man, I don't know. It feels like grasping for straws. Either way, it's not gonna happen over the weekend. By Monday, we'll have transferred him to Med-Psych for them to decide what to do."

Trey handed me the scrap paper where he had scribbled down the phone number of Scott's mom. Instead of calling her immediately, I looked online to read about medical causes for mania before I went back to writing my admission note on Scott. Then I took a bathroom break and scarfed down some snacks from the kitchen area. I was stalling. By that point of the year, I'd talked with family members of patients many times, and I'd never had a bad experience. More often, I valued these interactions, even when the patient had a serious—and sometimes fatal—condition. Comforting a family seemed part of a doctor's job. But in these cases, I had a better understanding of the illness the person faced, and I didn't have the emotional drain of a personal connection as I did with Scott.

When I returned to the medical floor, a nurse approached and told me that Scott's mother had called again. I couldn't delay any longer. I closed my eyes, took a deep breath, and picked up the scrap paper Trey had left. She answered on the first ring.

"Thanks for calling me back," she said.

I had braced myself for an entitled, professional-type parent, accustomed to getting things her way, angry that it had taken so long to get through to the doctor treating her son on the medical floor. But what I heard in her voice was gratitude. And fear.

"How is he doing now?" she asked, her breathing sounding as labored as if she had just jogged up several flights of stairs.

I thought about telling her that I knew Scott from years earlier. And that he was completely different from the person that I knew. "He's resting right now," I said instead.

I then relayed my conversation with Trey where we talked about what a medical workup might look like and how most of that couldn't be done until Monday.

"That's fine," she said. "Right now, I'm just happy the doctors in the emergency room listened to me and agreed to admit him to a medicine team and not a psychiatric unit."

"Where are you now?" I asked.

Her phone number had an out-of-state area code, which didn't mean as much with cell phone use beginning to become so widespread then. Still, I assumed that if she was local, we would have been sitting across each other in a family conference room.

"New York," she said. "That's where Scott grew up and where our family still lives. My husband is in Chicago this week for a business trip. He's coming back early from that tonight to watch our daughter, and I'm going to fly down there first thing in the morning."

She went on to explain that her daughter was a competitive junior soccer player and was playing in a high-level tournament that weekend. And that she had another daughter who was a sophomore at Cornell. It didn't feel like bragging to me. Instead, I suspected she offered some version of this family biography whenever she thought it necessary, in an attempt to prevent others from placing her kids in stereotypical racial boxes. With a tall, young-adult black son acting erratically in front of strangers hundreds of miles away, she probably felt that she needed to summon all the privilege at her disposal to soften their perception of him. She probably didn't realize, hearing my race-neutral-sounding voice, that she was speaking to someone who fully understood that worldview.

"I know that Scott went to college down here," I said. "But what is he doing now?"

"He started graduate school this semester," she answered. "In public health."

"Have you been in contact with him recently?" I asked.

She told me they'd last talked the previous week and he'd seemed distracted. She was a little concerned, but he sounded rational enough to ease her worries.

"The psychiatry resident in the emergency department told me that Scott has a history of depression treatment," I said. "When did that start?"

Scott's mom told me that he had gotten depressed during the spring semester of his junior year of college and had ended up taking a leave of absence.

"He hadn't been living right," she said.

"What do you mean?"

She said he had started smoking marijuana and eating poorly, and had gained twenty pounds. She'd set him up to see a psychiatrist in New York who prescribed three different antidepressant medications, one after the other, but none of them seemed to help much. What worked best, she said, was when Scott stopped smoking marijuana and started eating a clean diet. He returned to school and finished up his senior year with no major problems.

"When they called me last night," she said, "my first thought was that he had gone back to using that stuff. But they said his test came back negative. Do you know if it could be a false-negative result?"

She shared my hope that his behavior was somehow drug- or medication-related. We then spent a few minutes talking about possible medical causes for his behavior, as I ran through a list that included infections, endocrine disruptions, rheumatic illness, neurological problems, and metabolic diseases. While any of these diagnoses were possible, the overwhelming majority of people who develop manic or psychotic symptoms don't have any of these conditions. But we held out hope. It felt almost as if, in that moment, both his mother and I would have preferred that he have a brain tumor (one that wouldn't kill him, of course) than be diagnosed with some mysterious illness that no blood test or brain scan could identify. The sound of hoofbeats had us searching for a zebra when there were horses all around us.

"We're going to do everything we can," I said.

"Thanks so much. I really appreciate you talking with me like this."

My impression of her had changed radically from when I'd learned that Scott's lawyer-parents had brokered his admission to our medicine floor. What at first had seemed like snooty entitlement instead felt like his mom's desperation to cling to the railing as she fell down a flight of stairs. Of all the things that I had done that afternoon as an intern, dealing with life-and-death illness with several patients, this phone conversation stood out as the most difficult experience, physically and emotionally. But it was about to get worse.

Within moments of getting off the phone, I was jolted from my thoughts by screaming voices in the distance. Then a nurse's voice blared across the overhead speaker: "Code gray, eighth floor. Code gray, eighth floor."

Instinctively, I knew that this commotion involved Scott. I jumped from my seat and dashed toward his room, fearing what might await me.

TWO POLICE OFFICERS RAN PAST ME. OUTSIDE SCOTT'S ROOM, I saw a group of nurses and nursing assistants huddled, gawking at the scene. The only time it was like this was when a patient coded and staff administered CPR. At the nearby sink, I saw a nursing assistant being helped by another aide. They dabbed wet paper towels over her face, neck, and stained clothes.

"What happened?" I asked a nurse.

"The patient in there." She pointed to Scott's room. "He threw his food at her."

Because he'd been flagged as a "behavior risk," Scott had been assigned a nurse aide at his bedside, just like he had in the ER. This also meant he'd been given only paper and plastic items to consume his food. Still, a well-thrown milk carton, pudding cup, and large chocolate chip cookie could, at the very least, frighten a staff worker and raise worries that the patient might do even more down the line with his bare hands, injured or not.

I thought about Scott's threats to me, which I had been too embarrassed to admit to anyone. Maybe I should have told Trey and tried to prevent him from being admitted to our floor.

"Get away from me!" Scott screamed at the police officers, who now stood at the entrance to his room.

The police officers were in their thirties, thick-chested guys. They put on latex gloves. One of them spoke to Scott in a stern voice. "Here's the deal, young man. You can make this easy on yourself, or you can make it hard. It's your choice how this goes."

That kind of threat would have scared me into compliance, but they were trying to reason with someone who was irrational. Did they understand this? I was afraid that Scott might lash out at them and get himself hurt.

"Get away from me!" he yelled again.

The police officer looked back at a young doctor who, by virtue of being nearby when things started, was the de facto person in charge. It was Ramish. We'd overlapped in medical school, and he was now in his third year of residency. I hadn't seen him in a few years. He'd gained fifteen pounds and had a few new strands of gray. This doctor thing was aging him fast.

"What do you want to do?" one of the officers asked him.

Ramish turned to the lead nurse. "Whose team is he on?" he asked her.

I was getting ready to speak when I heard Trey's voice behind me. "It's us," he said. "What's going on?" he asked me.

I got tongue-tied. I should have told him about Scott's behavior in the emergency room. Before I could answer, Ramish interrupted, "He just hit one of our nurse assistants with his food. And his drink too. I saw the whole thing. You guys have to get him off our floor," he demanded. "He's a crazy person."

My chest tightened. Scott was not a real person to him. He was a diagnosis. He was a problem. Someone who was making Ramish's life difficult. It felt eerily similar to my medical school experiences at the state hospital. And likely Ramish's too.

"We're on it," Trey answered. He then looked over at the lead nurse. "Do you have Haldol and Ativan available?"

She nodded. She held two small bottles in one hand and a syringe in the other.

"Give him five and two, then," Trey said.

"Five" was the dose of Haldol, the antipsychotic medication. "Two" was the dose of Ativan, the sedative. The intent was to put Scott into a chemically induced slumber.

The two officers stood at the entrance to Scott's room. The nurse then returned with the syringe full of medication. "This is your last chance to do this peacefully," one of the officers said. "Otherwise, we'll have to hold you down, and none of us want that."

Memories of the state hospital flooded me again. These officers were meeting Scott for the first time. They had no sense of his intelligence, his athletic talent, his passion for social justice. Instead, he appeared to them to be an angry, young black man. The kind our society constantly shows on the news doing bad things to others and having bad things happen to them.

"Wait," I said, mobilized from my shock. I stepped past a few of the floor nurses and found myself standing next to the officers. "Let me talk to him."

The officers exchanged concerned looks. But then they stepped aside. I slowly entered the room and stopped about ten feet from Scott.

"Scott," I said. "It's me. Damon."

He looked confused, just like he had when he'd first seen me downstairs. I feared that he'd already forgotten our exchange in his altered mental state.

"Can you get me out of here?" Scott asked, seeming to recognize me again. "Please."

"Scott," I said. "You're not yourself right now."

"I'm fine," he fired back. " I just want to go home."

"I just spoke with your mom in New York," I said. "She's scared. She's coming down tomorrow to see you. Please do what they say. I don't want you to get hurt."

He scanned his surroundings. He was trapped. Still, I feared he'd lash out violently. And I would get hit first. What on earth had I done, trying to play hero? Nothing in my personality pointed to me acting like this. Despite my size, and the fear it sometimes evoked in others, the truth is that I was frequently afraid that others might hurt me.

But instead of Scott assaulting me, something clicked in his mind.

"I'll take the medicine," he said. "I'm sorry about what happened to that woman."

I looked away as the nurse gave him the medications. The cluster of medical staff dispersed back to their clinical duties, the same way they did after a CPR episode. The police officers waited a few minutes to make sure things remained calm.

"I think we gotta ship him over to psych ASAP," Trey said. "That workup his mom wants is gonna have to wait until later."

I couldn't hold in the truth any longer. I told Trey that I had played basketball with Scott many times when he was in college. Trey looked at me, first in disbelief, then with pained eyes. His face seemed to say that he understood and was sorry for what I'd just experienced.

I told him that I needed to get outside for fresh air. He nodded. I

wanted to clear my head before calling Scott's mother to update her. I'd
tell her that I knew Scott as more than what he was in that moment. I
imagined comforting her. But I worried I might fail miserably. Scott's
physical wounds would eventually heal, but what about his mind?

IN THE END, I DIDN'T CALL SCOTT'S MOTHER. TREY CONTACTED THE
psychiatry consult doctor on duty who saw Scott. She explained that
weekend transfers to psychiatric facilities, especially after Saturday mornings, were exceedingly hard to pull off due to staff-related issues and suggested that we instead start aggressively treating his psychiatric symptoms
while he was on our medical floor. Since he'd agreed to take medication,
she recommended valproic acid, an anti-seizure medication commonly
used in bipolar disorder, along with a daily antipsychotic drug. Her conversation with Trey was so clinical, so utterly detached. But maybe that
was required to get Scott what he needed in that moment. Before long,
I found myself entangled with the usual array of medical intern-type issues, patient A needing this treatment, patient B needing that test, and
so on. The pace didn't slow until the wee hours of Sunday morning. For
me, that was probably best.

When I returned to work that Monday morning after a sixteen-hour
break from the hospital, Scott had been transferred to the inpatient psychiatric unit. I didn't ask questions. Our patients that day had diabetes,
heart failure, lung infections, and the other usual problems seen on the
medical service. Like always, they were at different stages in the cycle
of admission, diagnosis, treatment, and discharge, and my job was to
keep track of each person in this perpetual chain. The only mention of
Scott came after we'd finished our preliminary morning rounds. As we
sat down in the workroom, Jason, the second-year resident who'd been
out sick on Saturday, looked over at me.

"I heard you had a crazy patient," he said. "Some real psych-ward stuff."

Jason sounded just like Trey when he'd gotten the initial call from the
ER. Just like Ramish when he'd told us we had to exile Scott far from
our medical floor. Just like me, until I'd seen he was Scott. From his tone,

I assumed he wasn't aware that Scott was someone that I'd personally known. Maybe Trey had decided it was best to keep that between me and him. I didn't have the emotional energy to open myself up to Jason.

"That's for sure," I said in reply. "It was rough going."

Our faculty supervisor arrived moments later to begin our formal teaching rounds for the day, and Scott's name never came up again. I could have called his mom, but I was no longer his doctor, I told myself. I could have contacted one of the psychiatry residents for an update, but it was easier to get lost in the daily grind of internship. And a lot safer. Seeing Scott as he'd been, and later talking with his mother, made me feel powerless and sad. I didn't want to stay too close to anything that evoked those emotions.

What I hadn't yet fully grasped though was how fragile the boundary could be between doctor and patient, between mentally well and mentally ill. As the internship year progressed, I saw these barriers become increasingly tenuous; a profession that held psychiatric education and practice at arm's length ironically had so many of its trainees and practitioners cracking under its own weight.

3

PROXIMITY

THE FOURTH TIME THE INTERN PAGED ME, I KNEW SOMETHING WASN'T right. Cara had paged me ten minutes earlier, and ten minutes before that, and ten minutes before that, each time asking for the blood test results needed to transfer a patient from my service to hers. But we had to wait for the central lab to enter those numbers into the data system; I had no way to get them any sooner than she could. I said as much to her each time, only it didn't seem to sink in.

I tried to be understanding. Internship year was grueling for us all, and this particular night, especially so for her. She was covering nearly twice as many patients as I was, and earlier in the evening, as we sat next to each other, I'd heard her pager blare a dozen times in less than five minutes. But later, my patience eroded when, even after the test result came back, and the patient was stable for transfer to her team, she paged me five more times when a single call would have sufficed. How could she get the work done on her massive checklist, I wondered, if she spent so much time calling me?

The strangeness of this encounter was still stuck in my mind a few nights later when I sat in a hospital conference room at midnight, scarfing down bad pizza with Evan, a fellow intern, and Joe, a senior resident who was supervising us for that shift. We'd been on duty over sixteen hours, with another dozen left. Despite us openly wishing we were someplace else at this hour of the day, we gravitated toward medical talk: how many patients were on our list, what kinds of problems they had, and so on. By the time we were on our second slice, I brought up my recent interaction with Cara, recounting her bizarre persistence in repeatedly paging me.

"Why was she doing that to you?" asked Evan. "That's so painful."

"I have no idea," I said as some of the frustration of that night returned in my mind.

"What's her name?" Joe asked.

Suddenly, I felt a twinge of regret. I didn't want to get her in trouble.

"It doesn't really matter, I guess," I replied, trying to change the subject. "It's over now."

Joe wasn't satisfied. He was my supervisor for the evening, and I had brought this concern to his attention; it didn't feel like I could refuse to answer. I leaned toward him and whispered her last name.

"I know who you're talking about," he said, his eyes widening with enthusiasm.

My guilt intensified. As much as I might enjoy listening to gossip, I hated spreading it. People's secrets were safe with me. I should have kept my mouth shut.

"I've interacted with her before," Joe continued. "She's wacky."

Joe described a time when he and Cara shared a patient in the emergency department, and the man confided to him that she had asked him the same questions over and over—so many times, the patient said, that the stomach pain that had brought him to the hospital had vanished, replaced by a big headache from hearing her voice.

Evan laughed hard. So did Joe. I chuckled nervously, still remorseful I'd mentioned her name, but also amused by Joe's description. Now, I wonder what was so funny. Was it a sexist, male-bonding ritual at the expense of this woman? Did it make us feel better about ourselves? I can't answer for their motives or, these many years later, for my own.

And then, we moved on. Evan started talking about an upcoming basketball game between Duke and his undergraduate school and how much he wanted to see Duke lose. The warning signs that something might be amiss with Cara blew right past us. As doctors, we were taught to recognize clinical patterns: a man gets short of breath while gardening one day and has left arm pain while biking the next week, and our training tells us to take a closer look at his heart. Had Cara experienced discrete physical symptoms like this, and they had come to our awareness, we would have been appropriately concerned.

Instead, she seemed to be exhibiting severe obsessive-compulsive behavior on at least two occasions. We'd seen those characteristics in patients, but the idea that a young doctor might suffer in that way seemed lost on us. Anyone, doctors included, could get struck down with an inflamed gallbladder or a bout of pneumonia, but only a "defective" person would be unable to get control of their thoughts and emotions. And as doctors, we had been told throughout our academic lives, and in turn told ourselves, that not only were we not defective, we were its opposite in every way. Thus, we chalked up Cara's behavior as being "wacky" in a difficult or annoying manner. The idea that we should be worried about her well-being or the patients under her care never came to the surface.

OUR INDIFFERENCE WAS ALL THE MORE ASTOUNDING—WELL, MINE was anyway—because by that point in my medical internship, just past the midpoint, I was seriously considering transferring from general medicine to psychiatry for the following year.

While my interaction with Scott months earlier had left me confused and helpless, it also made me acutely aware of the many overlaps between medical and psychiatric illness. Over the ensuing weeks after seeing Scott, I admitted several people whose medical problems—malnutrition from anorexia, possible liver failure from a Tylenol overdose, seizures from severe alcohol withdrawal—had a clear psychiatric basis. In the past, I would have eagerly passed off these psychiatric concerns to other doctors, but with Scott's breakdown in my mind, I wanted to learn more about what had brought these patients to our doorstep. I tried to envision them in an earlier, stabler place in life. In ways I never had before, I sought to understand my patients as people outside the hospital setting. So whenever time allowed, I listened intently to snippets about their lives, seeking clues to how things went awry. If I was not yet inching my way toward psychiatry, I was at least inching away from the prevailing medical view of psychiatric patients as people best kept at arm's length.

One case in particular triggered my interest in psychiatry, not because it revealed some great insights into humanity or a deep understanding of myself, but rather it showed me how a psychiatrist could be a "real doctor" in a medical crisis. Until then, while I knew that psychiatrists could help people break the grip of suicidal obsessions or psychotic thinking, I'd embraced the typical medical belief that they were basically useless for patients with acute physical problems. Mind and body were separate, to my thinking then, and patients facing urgent medical issues needed to have those concerns tamed first before psychiatrists could help. The culture of medical education that marginalized emotional health and psychiatrists had primed me to think this way. On an otherwise mundane weekday afternoon at the hospital, however, I discovered that I had been duped.

I had been called down to the emergency department to admit a woman with altered mental status, the same label Scott initially had. Only in this instance, Beth was in her late forties, and unlike Scott, her vital signs were askew. Her heart was pounding at a rate of about 150 beats per minute, well over the normal range for a healthy adult at rest. Her blood pressure was high too, checking in at a systolic level of 165 over a diastolic of 110. According to her sister, Beth had never had an issue with either. She also had a low-grade fever, her temperature hovering above 100 degrees.

"We don't know what the hell is going on," Dr. Lance, the emergency medicine physician, told Julie, the other doctor on my medical team upstairs, and me as we discussed her case in one of the physician workrooms. "But she definitely needs to be admitted."

The story they had thus far came from her sister, because Beth couldn't seem to talk. Her sister had gotten worried when Beth didn't answer her phone on a Sunday evening, and frightened when Beth hadn't shown up for work that Monday. She rushed over to Beth's house midday and found her alive, but in a trancelike state. She called 911.

"CT scan doesn't show a stroke or a tumor," Dr. Lance said. "Drug screen is clean."

"Anything on physical exam other than her abnormal vitals?" Julie asked.

"She's rigid," he replied, "both in her arms and legs."

My eager doctor brain rattled through possible diagnoses. Julie seemed to be on the same track. "Antipsychotic meds?" she asked.

Neuroleptic malignant syndrome is a rare condition we learned about in medical school most often caused by drugs used to treat schizophrenia and bipolar disorder. Abnormally stiff muscles and elevated vital signs were cardinal features. It was one of dozens of illnesses that we saw many more times on standardized tests than we did in real life.

"Far as we can tell, no history of those kind of drugs," Dr. Lance said as he shook his head. "Her sister says there is a history of depression and that she's been treated here in our psych clinic. But you know we can't see those damn notes."

At the time, the psychiatric service maintained an entirely different electronic medical record program from the one used by the rest of the hospital system, and access to it was restricted to those in their department. From what I knew, this was designed to maintain the privacy of their clients. Maybe you didn't want your dermatologist knowing that you had cheated on your wife, or have your knee surgeon reading about your sexual insecurities, the thinking went. The psychiatric medication list was the only thing that transferred to the general medical record, since other doctors had to know that information to avoid prescribing meds that might cause dangerous drug interactions. (This antiquated system remained for many years before becoming more modernized.)

"Prozac is on her med list," Dr. Lance continued, "but her sister thinks she stopped taking that more than a month ago."

That seemed to rule out serotonin syndrome, another condition often related to psychiatric drug use where people could become acutely confused. We had learned in textbooks and lectures that it could be caused by overdoses of various antidepressant pills.

"Maybe she's using some drug that doesn't show up on our screen?" Julie asked.

Dr. Lance nodded. "I called Psych to come see her so they can tell us what's in her psych chart. They're in with her now. But my bet is that this is all medical. When Psych is done, we're going to do an LP."

LP stands for *lumbar puncture*, also known as a *spinal tap*. Doctors stick a needle in the lower back to remove the fluid that bathes the spinal cord and brain. It's how we diagnose meningitis, multiple sclerosis, and various other neurological conditions.

Just as Julie and I were headed to see another patient in the emergency unit that we were admitting upstairs, the psychiatry resident entered the work area. He was tall, clean-shaven, with a hairline starting to recede. He looked past us and directly at Dr. Lance.

"She's got catatonia," he said without equivocation.

I thought about my medical school rotation at the state hospital. One afternoon, we watched a video recording about what state hospitals looked like in the 1950s that included scenes of patients with catatonia, a condition of unknown cause that impairs physical movement and responsiveness to the surrounding environment. In the clips, the people moved weirdly or not at all; they spoke bizarrely or were mute. I'd never seen anything like that in real life.

"Was there something in her chart about her having a history of it?" Julie asked.

The psych resident shook his head. "The chart just shows recent clinic treatment for depression. She missed her last two appointments and hasn't been seen in six months. About ten years ago, her depression was bad enough for her to be hospitalized."

"I thought catatonia was only in people with schizophrenia," Dr. Lance said.

"Actually, it's just as common with severe depression. Maybe even more so."

Dr. Lance and Julie shared a skeptical glance. But since the nuances of severe depression versus schizophrenia was "psych stuff," they didn't challenge his statement.

"But what about her fever, tachycardia, and hypertension?" Dr. Lance asked.

"Catatonia, when it's in a malignant state, like this, can present with unstable vital signs. She needs to get IV Ativan ASAP."

"But that's a sedative," Dr. Lance said as a frown spread across his face. "How is that supposed to help someone who is already bedbound?"

"No one knows for sure," the psych resident answered. "But if you don't believe me, call my attending. You can also find articles about it on MEDLINE."

The psych resident walked off without any parting pleasantries. I couldn't quite tell if he was socially awkward, or arrogant, or just busy and confident of his diagnosis.

"I'm not sure what to make of all that," Dr. Lance said, shaking his head. "But I'll look into what he said and let you both know."

Julie and I went to see Beth in her treatment room. She was alone. The top of her bed was inclined to about thirty degrees. She had a blood pressure cuff around her fleshy upper-left arm and a pulse oximeter device on her right index finger. Up close, her brown hair and olive complexion were grimy; it appeared she'd gone days without washing. Her eyes were open, but they didn't follow us as we approached. Other than involuntary eye blinking and the slight rise and fall of her chest, she was still. Completely still.

"Hello," I said to her. "Can you hear us?"

No response. Julie tapped Beth's arm, then her shoulder, and finally her neck. She never budged. Julie tried to lift her arm at the elbow, but Beth seemed to resist while otherwise remaining still.

"It must have taken three nurses to change her and get her all hooked up," I said.

Everything about how Beth looked in that moment seemed unnatural. As if she were purposefully faking her sickness for some reason we had yet to discover. But how could she fabricate a fever, high blood pressure, and a rapid heart rate?

I soon got busy with calls from upstairs, and two hours passed before I saw Beth again. On the way to the ER work area to get an update from

Dr. Lance, I nearly tripped as I glanced into her room. Beth was sitting up. Her arms were moving. She was sipping water.

A younger woman, heavyset, with long black hair, stood next to her bed, helping Beth steady the water glass. I approached the room.

"Are you the psych doctor?" the woman eagerly asked.

"No. I'm one of the doctors upstairs—"

"Well, I want to see him," she interrupted. "I was gone when he came by."

"Are you a family member?" I asked.

"I'm her sister," she replied. "I'm the one who called 911. I'm sorry I had to leave but I had to take my son to a doctor's appointment. He's got bone cancer."

I tried to imagine the stress of finding her sister unresponsive that morning while navigating her son's cancer treatment. I couldn't.

"If he's left," she continued, "please thank him. The nurse said he suggested giving her this drug, Ativan, and look at her, it's working."

I looked at the digital monitors. Her pulse and blood pressure were still elevated but had lowered. I turned to Beth. Her eyes met mine. She slowly pulled her mouth away from the drinking straw. It looked as if she was trying to smile or even speak, but she hadn't fully escaped the grasp of whatever had frozen her.

Moments later, I walked up to Dr. Lance in the nearby physician work area. He saw me approaching from Beth's room.

"I'll be damned," he said. "That psych resident was right. I read up on catatonia. It's freakin' amazing. We use Ativan down here all the time to knock out violent and psychotic people, and somehow it also works on someone who wasn't moving at all. That's crazy."

I shared his astonishment. I'd seen medications rapidly treat heart arrhythmias and antibiotics obliterate infections, but nothing like this in psychiatry. The closest were drugs that blunted the symptoms of alcohol withdrawal, but the results weren't this dramatic.

"She still needs to be admitted, though, right?" I asked.

He nodded. "From what I'm reading, she'll need to keep getting dosed with Ativan for a while. Still has a ways to go, but without treatment, it sounds like she would have ended up in really bad shape."

Catatonia can in some cases progress to a malignant state where the body's automatic processes that control body temperature, heart rate, and blood pressure become so dysregulated that it can ultimately cause irreversible damage and even death. Beth, with her abnormal vital signs, may have been on that path had we not intervened.

We admitted Beth to our medical floor overnight, where she improved further. The next morning, we contacted the Med-Psych service, a team of rotating doctors who dealt with complex cases where the two disciplines overlapped. They agreed to take Beth.

Later that morning, I saw Dr. Colter, the lead doctor on their team that week, alone in a physician workroom. She was midthirties, probably only five years or so ahead of me professionally, but that felt like an eternity. I hesitantly approached her.

"I admitted that woman with catatonia yesterday," I began. "That was incredible to see how much better she got after getting Ativan. None of us in the ED could believe it."

She smiled. "The mind-body interface is fascinating."

I thought back to my research experience as a third-year medical student. The many articles I'd read about how emotional stress affected the physical body. How this basic concept had been known for centuries but its specifics were still not well understood. Some medical students are attracted to the hands-on part of medicine: cutting out tumors, fixing broken bones, repairing ruptured blood vessels. Others find the mystery of disease more appealing: the various ways it can announce itself throughout the body, the diagnostic process of solving the puzzle, the use of medications and other treatments to counteract these aberrations. Over time, I discovered that I felt more at home with this latter group. And as mysteries went, the brain stood apart, not only for how it housed our thoughts and our emotions but also the many ways in which it controlled the physical body.

"Do you see a lot of interesting cases like this in your work?" I asked. "You know, from the psych side?"

She looked at me curiously. "Sure, from my standpoint, I do. Most aren't quite this dramatic, though."

I told her that at the state hospital I'd seen how psychiatric care could be useful to people with schizophrenia or suicidal depression, but not how that knowledge could be directly helpful in treating patients with serious general medical conditions.

"Do you think you might be interested in psych or med-psych?" she asked.

I started to reflexively say *no*, the same *hell no* reply if she'd just asked me to sing karaoke in front of the nurses on the medical floor. But something stopped me. The perplexing nature of mental illness had gradually become appealing after my early months of internship, and the amazing incident with Beth amplified those feelings. Still, in that moment, I was training to become a "real doctor," and medicine's disrespect for psychiatry had been deeply ingrained. So before answering her question, I got up and closed the door so our conversation remained private.

"Maybe," I said. "I'm not sure what I'm thinking right now."

It was the first time I'd said that out loud. It felt exciting and confusing all at once. I'd started medical residency with the intent to become a cardiologist. I enjoyed reading EKGs, listening to heart sounds with my stethoscope, and viewing heart anatomy and function on echocardiograms. But I had little interest in the procedural parts of the field—catheterizations, stents, and ablations—and those areas seemed to be what was increasingly driving innovation and prestige within the field. I was ambivalent about spending another six years in training to become what I worried might be a second-class cardiologist.

Dr. Colter eyed the closed door. "Well, if you're thinking about transferring into psych, I understand that you might be concerned with how your colleagues will perceive you. That you're crazy or not as smart as they are. It was like that where I went to med school."

She'd read my mind. Before I could ask how she had gotten over any feelings of inadequacy, she connected psychiatry to other doctors in a way I had never considered.

"But as one of our psychiatrists on faculty here likes to say," she continued, "other doctors look down on psychiatrists until they or someone they love needs one, and a lot of them end up needing one."

Really? I thought. While the COVID-19 pandemic has brought into the public domain broader awareness of high burnout rates, clinical depression, impairing anxiety, and substance misuse rates among health care workers of all stripes, the many doctors trained during a time when such topics were mentioned in whispered passing. I didn't know back then that psychiatric illness was especially common among medical students and physicians. I'm not sure I would have believed it in any case. Weren't we too exceptional for such human failings, acing test after test from grade school onward, on a path to saving lives and making lots of money? That was certainly the story many of us had told ourselves for a long time.

My pager went off, signaling that it was time to get back to work.

"Thanks for talking to me," I said. "Please don't tell anyone that we talked. I don't want any rumors—"

She held up her hand to stop my babbling. "Sure thing," she said with a smile. "Generally, those of us in psych are pretty good with that."

Dr. Colter told me I could reach out to her at any time if I had questions. She also encouraged me to contact the psychiatry training director. Weeks went by, and I did neither; a busy month in the ICU had me revert back to survival mode. Then the incident with Cara happened—the excruciating hours of her constantly paging me, the subsequent laughs at her expense with my colleagues over pizza. But I didn't initially make the connection between her behavior and Dr. Colter's admonition of how prevalent mental illness was among doctors. More weeks passed, until one afternoon I picked up the phone to call Dr. Colter.

Earlier that day, I'd completed the medical history and physical exam on a sixtysomething man who'd come to the hospital after passing out at home. Although he had been recently diagnosed with diabetes and high blood pressure, the EMTs on the scene found him in the opposite state: hypoglycemic and hypotensive. He was so afraid of having a stroke or needing dialysis, his wife told me, that he'd begun checking his blood glucose and blood pressure numbers every hour throughout the day, and taking more of his diabetes and anti hypertensive meds than his doctor had prescribed. He couldn't "turn off his brain," his wife said. This obsessive-compulsive pattern, with his preoccupation on medical data, triggered me to think of Cara.

I rehearsed what I'd say to Dr. Colter: I would tell her that I'd interacted with a fellow intern a few weeks earlier whom I suspected was in need of psychiatric treatment. Could she help me find someone to reach out to her?

But just before my finger punched the first digit of Dr. Colter's pager number, I pulled the receiver back from my ear and held it suspended in the air, midway between my head and the base of the desktop phone. The monotonous dial tone hummed, awaiting my action. Finally, it grew impatient and the buzz became a blaring disconnect signal that jarred me from my trance. I quickly hung up the phone to silence it.

I couldn't make the call. As an intern, I was responsible for doing whatever I could to help patients in need. But when the person in need was another doctor, that impulse felt like the equivalent of a meddling kid tattling on his classmate. And for what purpose? Sure, Cara had annoyed the hell out of me, but the patient we'd shared had been unharmed. Maybe we had crossed paths on her absolute worst day at work, and she was otherwise a great intern. But then I thought about what my senior resident said about his encounter with her in the emergency room, where she kept repeating the same questions to a patient they treated. Two episodes separated in time and space—that was our foundation in suspecting the diagnosis of multiple sclerosis for people with vague neurological symptoms. Common sense suggested the same might be true for identifying a troubled mind, no matter whose mind it might be.

I toyed with the idea of calling Cara myself, or waiting until the next time I saw her around the hospital to express my concerns. But how would she take "I'm worried about you" from someone she didn't know? I couldn't envision a positive outcome. What if she broke down? Then what? I also worried that I might jeopardize her career if other people found out I had pointed her in the direction of Dr. Colter. I was too busy with my own life to get that involved in someone else's. Besides, I told myself, if what I'd seen and heard was part of a larger issue, someone else in her daily workspace would notice it and act. Although I was ashamed at laughing about her with colleagues, ultimately, I decided, the health of a colleague was not my problem.

TWO MONTHS AFTER MY ENCOUNTER WITH CARA, I SAT DOWN FOR lunch with Greg, a fellow intern. My initial guilt, and subsequent impulse to contact Dr. Colter for guidance to help her, had both faded as internship year wore on. Although I was inching toward choosing psychiatry, I still maintained a vast disconnect between what I thought of the field in theory and the people that it impacted in reality. Greg and I devoured our greasy meals within a few minutes, as the food momentarily quelled the tensions of intern life. We talked about college basketball before the conversation turned serious.

"How have you been doing?" he asked, his eyes locking with mine.

He wasn't asking simply to make small talk. I sensed that he was either concerned about me or wanted to share details about himself. Or both.

"Tired," I said, honestly. "It's been a long year."

"I hear you on that," he replied. "Sometimes I wonder, you know, if it's all worth it in the end. But maybe that's on my mind right now because of what I heard this morning."

"What?" I asked.

One of our colleagues had told him about a fellow intern who had an emotional breakdown in front of a patient and ended up making a mistake. As he provided more details—scant as they were—I felt the muscles in my neck clench and my heart flutter. The doctor he described was the very same intern who had paged me over and over, hour upon hour, one evening about the results of a blood test. The same one I and two other doctors had laughed about a few nights later. The same one I had later thought needed treatment but decided not to get involved with. Cara.

"I don't know all the details," Greg said, as I began peppering him with questions. "They were able to correct whatever mistake she made with the patient."

"That's good news," I said. "Really good news."

"But it looks like there is no way that she's going to be able to stay around."

My mind flashed back to the single day we worked together, shortly before she started paging me nonstop. We sat in a physician/nurse workspace, writing orders in medical charts. Cara seemed tense, anxious, stressed as she fielded one pager call after another. But no worse or different from other interns or residents I'd seen. I didn't think anything was unusual until later, when the flood of pages started.

Had she experienced emotional problems in medical school, or even earlier in life, I now wondered, that recurred or rapidly worsened under the crushing weight of internship? If so, did any of her supervisors know about her past? In the throes of that arduous year myself, I found it safer to focus on her possible limitations than to interrogate the sanity of the training system itself, where we normalized thirty-hour hospital shifts for brand-new doctors, often with little or no support. Questioning that structure too much would have meant casting doubt on my choice to attend medical school in the first place.

"You know," Greg began as he looked away. "What's that expression, 'There but for the grace of God, go I'? I'm not super religious or anything, but I mean, if I hadn't got back into treatment, maybe that could have been me."

"Treatment?" I said, confused at first. "What kind?"

Greg looked at me as if a teacher had unexpectedly called his name during class. He'd revealed more than he wanted.

"Sorry," I said. "You don't have to tell me anything."

He took in a short, deep breath and leaned in closer to me. "No, it's okay. I'll tell you. Between us. During my second year of medical school, I got pretty depressed. Nothing like that had ever happened to me before. I couldn't function."

I sat stunned. By this point in training, I'd seen depressed patients and had even written a handful of prescriptions. But the ones I'd encountered were mostly middle-aged and older, and medically sick or, in the few cases with younger patients, they had already faced years of deprivation of one sort or another. To my understanding at the time (naive as it sounds now), people dealing with depression were not doctors and dentists and professors, or any other well-educated people with prospects for good income and intellectually fulfilling jobs. As if being smart and economically well-off, attributes I highly valued, somehow insulated you from becoming depressed.

"I started seeing a therapist and got on Lexapro, and that really helped me out a lot," Greg continued. "I weaned off Lexapro the last year-plus of medical school and I felt fine. Things were good. But I started back on it around Thanksgiving after working in the ICU. That month was torture. I was starting to backslide. But I'm doing better now."

From my time at the state hospital and after my ordeal with Scott, I truly believed that schizophrenia and bipolar disorder were biological illnesses. But depression? Sure, some people got so bad that they became suicidal, but working in a hospital meant I saw people who developed serious medical problems that devastated their lives. Or, in the case of the patients at the state hospital, people who had experienced some horrible psychological trauma. In the absence of those conditions, depression seemed like something for people who just had trouble coping with the ups and downs of life, and, to paraphrase my grandmother, needed to get themselves together. Having built so many categories to wall myself off from seriously thinking about mental health issues, I didn't know what to make of what Greg had told me.

"Well," I stumbled. "I'm glad you're feeling better."

"Thanks for listening to me," he responded, looking at his watch and realizing he had to get back to work. "I'd greatly appreciate it if you kept this between us."

I told him that I would, just as Dr. Colter had given me a similar assurance regarding my interest in psychiatry. Over the next several days, I replayed this conversation with Greg, the sad ordeal with Cara, my secret discussion with Dr. Colter, Beth's miraculous recovery from catatonia, and Scott's shocking episode of mania and psychosis. I also thought about all the daily interactions I'd had with patients those last several months, and my growing interest in learning about them and their family members as people, rather than as a collection of diseased organs and body parts. Without fully recognizing it as such, a tug-of-war had been taking place inside me between the impulses drawing me toward psychiatry and the powerful forces resisting that change.

One morning, without any conscious trigger, I got tired of this internal struggle. I emailed the psychiatry training director and expressed my interest in transferring into the psychiatry program. She replied within the hour, and a few days later, I sat in her office. The following week, I met with some other psychiatry faculty, and just like that, I was offered a position as a psychiatry resident starting that July. All that was left was for me to tell my general medicine supervisors about my plans and power through the last three months of medical internship. Filled with renewed enthusiasm, I was confident that these weeks would be challenging but manageable; instead, I soon faced the most humbling and humiliating moments of my professional career.

MY TRANSFER DATE TO PSYCHIATRY WAS SET. ALL I HAD TO DO WAS keep a steady hand and an even keel as I'd done so far that year, and the process would proceed smoothly. But as I hunched over Ernest's enormous belly on a muggy Tuesday evening, needle in hand, sweating, aching, and swearing, I worried that I might not make it to the end.

Ernest, mid-fiftyish, had once led a functional life, operating a landscaping business and raising three kids with his wife. But in the aftermath of 9/11, he found himself having graphic nightmares about his military combat in Vietnam. He tried psychiatric medicines and group therapy, but they didn't help. Before long, the half dozen beers he'd drank daily for years became a dozen. And then his life fell apart. His business went under. His wife left him. Twelve beers became eighteen, and eighteen became a full case. What he did not know at the time was that his liver was already failing, and the extra alcohol accelerated its demise. When he came to us, he had severe cirrhosis and perhaps its most visible landmark: a protuberant abdomen filled with fluid that did not belong there.

The purpose of his admission was to remove some of this fluid, through a medical procedure called a *paracentesis*, and to adjust his medications so that he could breathe better and be in less pain. Ernest arrived on our floor around five o'clock in the evening. By then, our team had already admitted six new patients from the emergency room, one right after another, the floodgates having opened that morning after a weekend snowstorm had kept patients at home and ground normal hospital operations to a halt. In a year filled with busy day after busy day, this was perhaps the most suffocating one of all.

I entered Ernest's room along with Steven, a second-year medical resident a year ahead of me on the hospital hierarchy, and Miles, a medical student a few years my junior.

"Are you ready, sir?" Steven asked Ernest.

"Yes," Ernest said, rubbing his calloused hands over his bloated, discolored belly. "Get as much of this shit off as you can."

Steven and I had already decided that I would be the one doing the paracentesis, since he had done plenty so far during residency, while I needed to perform a certain number and variety of procedures to complete internship. This was my first paracentesis in the lead, but I had done the chest cavity equivalent: thoracentesis—a technically more difficult and potentially dangerous procedure—three times without any problem. I'd also placed central lines in large veins in the groin and neck, drawn arterial blood to assess blood oxygenation levels, and become proficient at getting routine blood samples when the phlebotomy staff was unavailable. Although I didn't enjoy this part of medicine as much as the cerebral side, I had steady hands. So I started things with Ernest thinking that it would go just fine.

I began by using medicated cotton swabs to sterilize the surface of his skin. I then gave him a topical anesthetic in the area where I planned to insert the tube. With little problem, I placed the pointed rubber tubing into an area where I thought fluid would flow freely. But when I attached the tube to the suction device, nothing came out, save for a few drops of blood.

"Damn," I said, as I felt beads of sweat collect in my armpits and across my brow.

"Try repositioning it," Steven told me.

I moved the white tubing clockwise, and then counterclockwise, but nothing came out. "You'll have to take it out and try again," Steven said.

I opened another needle and tubing set. Steven and I found a location we thought would be fruitful, but the result was the same. I'd failed twice. The trickle of perspiration was now a full-fledged sweat. "This is bullshit," I suddenly heard myself say aloud.

Steven's eyes widened. "Damon, you need to chill out, man."

"I'm fine," I said. I then looked up at Ernest. "Sorry about that."

"Just get it right the next time," he responded.

I was not okay. Maybe surgeons and anesthesiologists can get away with cursing and complaining when their patients are unconscious, but no doctor treating a patient at the bedside has that luxury. By any objective standard, Ernest's life was in far worse shape than mine, but in that moment, I felt like he and his distended belly were torturing me.

"Let me take it from here," Steven insisted.

He removed his white coat. Underneath, he wore a size-too-small scrub top that revealed thick biceps.

"I'm sorry," I said to him and to Ernest.

"Go get started on the other new patients. Take the student with you. I'll be done here in a few minutes and will catch up with you."

Without another word, I quickly gathered my things and rushed back to the workroom. Miles tagged behind. I kept my head down, fearing others could look into my eyes and see my shame. When I entered the workroom and found it empty, I exploded.

"This is fucking bullshit," I said as I hurled my clipboard across the room, sending papers sprawling in every direction.

I instantly regretted my behavior. I never could have imagined acting this way in any professional situation, let alone in the company of a medical student who I was supposed to mentor. But there was no way to undo my words and actions.

"I'm sorry," I said to Miles.

"It's okay," he said. "My sister is an intern at UNC, and she is struggling too."

Everything was backward. I was supposed to be giving him advice and encouragement, not the other way around.

"I just need to get something to eat and I'll feel better," I said, as I stormed off.

I went through the remainder of the evening and overnight shift in a mental haze. I couldn't believe I'd lost control in front of a patient and my colleagues. I'd never done anything like that. Not once. Steven and Miles didn't mention to me what had happened in Ernest's room or its immediate aftermath. Still, I worried that someone—I wasn't sure exactly who—might have overheard or seen my outburst, or would hear about it secondhand, and report me to a supervisor. With that fear, the next morning I preemptively went to the office of Dr. Thompson, the chief resident then, to confess my sins.

"I made a mistake," I said, barely able to look at him.

I explained what occurred and told him I understood if I needed to face some type of disciplinary action.

"There's no reason to punish you," he said. "But you might need some help."

I felt a tingle in the back of my head. "What . . . what do you mean?"

He sat back in his chair as he pulled at some of the hairs on his beard. "With you planning to go into psychiatry, you certainly know how important mental health is."

My chest and neck muscles tightened. Was he saying that I was crazy? Dr. Thompson and all the faculty leadership had been supportive when I'd told them weeks earlier of my decision to switch into psychiatry. Suddenly, it felt like he was using that against me.

"I think you should talk with someone from employee assistance before returning to work," he continued. "It sounds like you are in a rough place."

Once again, I had missed the point about mental health, only this time, I was the "patient." After my fit of fury, I had not tried to figure out what caused my reaction but instead focused on a single technical point: my inability to do the procedure. I'd come to the chief resident's office expecting that my "penance" would involve taking an extra shift or spending remedial time to ensure that I was competent to perform paracenteses. That outcome would have fit the model of medical training centered on memorization, technique, and repetition, rather than less tangible markers of performance and well-being. It's ridiculous to think about now, but the last thing I expected was to be told that I needed to see a therapist. Although I had committed to training in psychiatry, to my thinking at the time, this outcome felt like true punishment.

I started to protest. But as I took in his words and thought about my life, tears flooded my eyes. I was horrified. Since grade school, I could count on one hand the number of times I had cried: the night of my worst basketball game in high school, a car accident that could have proved fatal, the morning of my grandmother's death. That was it.

Why was I crying to Dr. Thompson? As best I could tell, it was a culmination of nine months of near-continuous sleep deprivation, the expectation of navigating life-and-death situations, and the endless pressure not to screw anything up that could hurt someone. And I'd just failed in that regard, even if Ernest suffered no major complications from my errors.

Dr. Thompson said he would speak to our program director immediately and arrange to give me time off. He tried to assure me these sort of mandated evaluations were not unusual, but I didn't believe him. I had botched a procedure, cursed about it, then cried about it, rather than just "man up" and soldier through the remaining months of internship.

At that moment, I felt like a complete failure; I had let down my patients, my colleagues, and everyone who had helped me to become a doctor in the first place.

THOUGH THE EMOTIONS THAT OVERWHELMED ME THAT DAY FELT LIKE mine alone, in fact they are pervasive within medicine. During medical school, I witnessed troubling episodes of dysfunctional behavior among doctors. One surgeon threw a temper tantrum and sharp instruments when the junior doctor and scrub nurse did not anticipate his needs in the OR. An OB-GYN resident ripped out pages from a patient's medical chart because the intern had made one error in his note. A medical resident slammed his pager against the wall when it kept going off during a busy afternoon. But these doctors all had their apologists, who asserted that their colleagues were "good" people who had the occasional "bad day" from the stress of their jobs. At the time, it had seemed like excuse-making for people with poor self-control. Until I found myself on the other side.

Why are physicians so vulnerable to bouts of emotional distress? Is it our own grinding competitiveness, which serves us well as premeds and medical students, but less so in the flesh-and-blood reality of clinical practice? Or is it a by-product of the culture of medicine itself, which values mental fortitude in the face of disease and death, and where displays of vulnerability are often seen as a sign of weakness?

To help me better understand this question, I spoke with Dr. Caroline Elton, a London-based psychologist with more than two decades of experience counseling physicians and medical students, and author of the 2018 book *Also Human: The Inner Lives of Doctors*. Dr. Elton sees the problem as more about systems than individual doctors.

"Everyone has their limit of what they can emotionally withstand," she told me, "and medical training has often historically failed to acknowledge that doctors are people too."

She noted the enduring struggle that new doctors face as they cope with the brutal transition from medical school, as well as the burdens on established physicians, who confront demands to see more patients in the midst of staff shortages and increasing bureaucratic tasks, rendering them unable to treat patients in the ways that attracted them to medicine in the first place. In both instances, doctors too often feel like they are suffering without support. She sees these circumstances as a recipe for work dissatisfaction and, ultimately, burnout.

But many physicians face even more worrisome struggles. Doctors are at least as likely to misuse alcohol as the average person and more likely to misuse prescription sedatives. During our training, we are more prone to episodes of depression than our age-matched peers. Most worrisome of all, doctors consistently have suicide rates that exceed the general population's. Each year, stories trickle out from training programs of residents who've died from suicide. Clearly, life as a physician can have bad side effects. The COVID-19 pandemic, it seems, made all of this even worse.

In those with more severe emotional distress, Dr. Elton believes that being proactive and vigilant can mitigate the worst outcomes.

"Typically, there are warning signs," she told me. "The issue is how we can support people better in the transition from medical school to internship. A new doctor might not want people in their training program knowing about their prior mental health struggles, but it can be immensely helpful if there is someone who can look out for them and support them."

Dr. Elton's book offers examples of doctors who benefited from the assistance that she and others provided. But others suffer in silence. This reluctance some doctors show to acknowledge health problems—both mental and physical—has hindered too many from seeking help. I knew this perspective well from personal experience, as it took much of medical school to accept that I had high blood pressure. If I was ashamed to acknowledge something so comfortably "medical," how much harder might it be to admit to a mental health problem? Add to this stubbornness the concern that medical information—especially mental health records—might go into one's permanent record with a hospital or state medical board, and it is not hard to envision a doctor turning to alcohol or prescription drugs—the latter readily at our disposal—rather than professional care. With my outburst, I had joined the ranks of the many healers in need of healing.

BASED ON MY CONVERSATION WITH DR. THOMPSON, I WAS REQUIRED to have an evaluation through the employee health service before I could return to the hospital wards. What I faced was strictly by the book. Still, I protested at first, offering to continue without a break, worried how this might impact the rest of my time in internal medicine and my transfer into psychiatry. But Dr. Thompson held firm as he tried to assuage my fears by insisting that the entire process would remain confidential.

I realized then that further protest would only make me seem more unstable. Whatever label one put on my mental state, I had to acknowledge that temporarily, at least, I was impaired.

I had never been to a counselor of any kind before. The location was thankfully a three-story building with a variety of offices rather than a designated mental health clinic. Nonetheless, I pulled the hood of my jacket over my head as I walked toward the entrance, just as a cheating spouse might on the way to a clandestine rendezvous.

But I pushed back the hood as I entered the building, lest I be mistaken for a mugger. Inside, I avoided eye contact with people as I scurried up the stairs to the third floor instead of waiting in the lobby for the elevator. Taking a deep breath, I opened the door and approached the check-in area, my shoulders hunched, my head down. A middle-aged clerk looked up.

"Can I help you?" she asked me.

"I have an appointment," I said as I quickly surveyed the small waiting area. There were a few other people there, none I recognized.

"What's your name?"

I showed her my badge to avoid saying my name aloud. She frowned. If the purpose of this appointment was to demonstrate my mental fitness, I was off to a bad start.

"Please have a seat. Someone will be with you shortly."

I sat in the farthest corner away from everyone and buried my face into a sports magazine. About five minutes later, a man's voice softly called my name: "Damon Tweedy."

I scanned the room, as if I were some celebrity whose visit to a counseling center might become tabloid fodder. But that fear quickly passed. The others in the waiting area were out of hearing range and, in any case, seemed too absorbed with their own problems to care about mine.

"Peter," the man said as we shook hands.

Until that moment, I had no idea who would be evaluating me. My counselor was five nine at most, with graying hair and thick eyebrows. He wore a brown sweater with a collared blue shirt underneath. I stole a glance at his employee badge; he was a licensed clinical social worker, not a psychiatrist or psychologist. Back then, I was unaware that social workers did this work, and was uncertain whether this distinction mattered. What had he been told about me?

On the short walk to his office, I suddenly became conscious of the racial dynamics. Black residents are more likely to face professional disciplinary issues, including getting kicked out of their training programs. I was about to enter the office of a middle-aged white man who, in that moment, seemed to have an outsize influence over what happened next with my medical career.

Once we were seated, he wasted no words getting to the heart of the matter.

"Your supervisor requested that you come speak with me."

I scanned the room, which, with its generic furniture and desktop computer, gave no signs of being a pseudo-confessional where people shared their secrets and shames. I was reluctant to speak, but recognized silence wasn't the way to convey robust mental health.

"I had a really bad day that day," I said.

He asked for details. I recounted the series of events that led to my eruption. I then explained how I prided myself on being competent and calm, and, in that moment, I was neither, in plain view of others. I talked about how tired I was from the year and how I looked forward to being finished.

"Residency is especially toxic," he responded. "I've been doing this for over ten years, and I've seen more residents come through here than anyone else."

I gave a half smile. While by this point I now knew that other doctors struggled too, it didn't stop me from feeling defective, carrying the irrational belief that my problems were mine alone. It was good to hear someone tell me that it wasn't all my fault. We agreed that my impending switch to psychiatry probably added to the grind of my remaining months of general medicine internship.

From there, we discussed how I'd decided to become a doctor, where I'd grown up, my hopes for the future. He reminded me how much I had already accomplished and that while I had experienced a clear setback, such events were often small blips in the arc of a career. He spoke positively about his work as a therapist, which in turn made me feel better about my choice to switch to psychiatry.

During a break in our conversation, I looked at my watch and realized that nearly forty-five minutes had passed.

"What happens next?" I asked.

I assumed that I'd "passed" the evaluation, just as I'd passed other tests I'd encountered in my life, but still I wanted my official "grade." In my view, it felt like I should receive a "good-conduct A." I didn't drink alcohol or use drugs. I wasn't suicidal or delusional. During our session, I hadn't broken down sobbing uncontrollably, nor had I cursed or been confrontational in any conceivable way. I'd been a "good" patient.

"I'll send my report to employee health," he said. "And they'll be in touch with your program director."

The mention of a "report" raised alarms in my head. I knew it wouldn't end up in my general medical chart, which for me included doctors' visits for sprained ankles, back problems, high blood pressure, and eye exams. But what about in the separate psychiatric electronic file? Would I be permanently branded as a psych patient?

"No, this will exist strictly outside our electronic recordkeeping," he assured me.

I wanted to ask more questions about the paperwork, but recognized he couldn't give an answer that would fully alleviate all my concerns.

The next morning, a Thursday, Dr. Thompson called and instructed me to take off the remainder of that week, with clearance to return to work the following Monday. When I walked back in the hospital that humid morning, I had been away less than a week, but in some ways I felt as refreshed as if I'd taken an extended vacation. During my brief hiatus, I exercised, slept, and ate home-cooked meals. I watched *Law & Order* reruns and read a novel. What had started out an experience of feeling punished and singled out had turned into a respite where I was left feeling . . . almost restored. In Dr. Elton's analysis, based on the many doctors she'd counseled in her London-based setting, I had experienced burnout, but my robust response to the time off work suggested that I had not been depressed.

My next rotation took place on a wing of the hospital where I had never worked. The patients, nurses, and doctors were new. It was a fresh start. Toward the end of that first week, I ran into Andrew, a fellow intern, on my way from the hospital cafeteria. We had been friendly during a rotation together earlier in the year after discovering shared interests in football and the *Godfather* movie franchise.

"How is everything going, Damon?" he asked.

It was an innocent enough question, the mundane kind we ask one another every day without really caring about the answer. But Andrew's eyes gave me their undivided attention. I sensed he'd caught wind of what happened to me, but I was not about to tip my hand. "Not too bad," I said. "Same as always."

He quickly cut through my veneer. "I covered for you last week."

I retreated a half step and quickly scanned our perimeter. I feared other interns or residents were within earshot, but thankfully, none were. Until then, I had no idea who replaced me on the medical service, nor had I given it any thought. I'd been called as one-week backup myself a few months earlier, to fill in for a colleague whose wife had delivered their first child—so in pure math terms, I had put more into the system than I'd taken out. Nevertheless, my knees wobbled as I stood next to Andrew. The cafeteria tray suddenly became unsteady in my hands; Coke dribbled down the side of the Styrofoam cup.

"I'm sorry you had to fill in for me," I said. "I can't thank you enough."

"No worries," he replied. "We're all in this together. I'm just glad you're back."

I smiled to keep from crying, moved by his graciousness and genuine concern. Too often, it seemed, there was very little of those sentiments to go around in the busy world of the hospital.

I thought about Cara. What if one of her colleagues or supervisors—if *I*—had stepped in to help before it was seemingly too late? Or maybe someone had tried, and still her problems proved too severe to survive life in medicine as it operated then. I suspected, however, that everyone else had done what I did and made excuses for leaving her alone. Until she crashed and burned.

WOULD THINGS HAVE BEEN DIFFERENT FOR CARA HAD SHE TRAINED in our current times?

I posed this question to Dr. Aimee Zaas, the current director of the internal medicine residency at Duke, the same program where I'd started two decades earlier.

"Things are a lot different on these issues than when you and I trained," she told me.

Dr. Zaas described a variety of structural changes that reduced work hours, allowed greater flexibility with vacation days, and sought to achieve a better balance between intensive clinical rotations and less grueling ones. But equally important, she said, was something less tangible.

"There has been a culture shift in how people in medicine are approaching mental health. It has become more acceptable to talk about and to address. Not only would she have had more resources available to help her from the outset, but if you or I were residents now, we would be more likely to be proactive in trying to get her help."

I thought back to internship year. During our orientation week, some faculty person—I can't remember who—mentioned to us that psychological stress was common for interns. But I don't recall being given details of confidential services where people could self-refer for counseling. That information would have been valuable, not only at the outset, but throughout the year as challenges mounted. If we'd all had a referral source handy, we probably would have been more likely to have sat down with Cara, rather than avoiding her or mocking her.

As for the future, I hope Dr. Zaas is right. But the continued reports of emotional suffering among doctors, heightened during COVID-19, make me worry that even though certain facets of addressing physician wellness have changed for the better, others remain intractable.

Perhaps there is something about us, as doctors, that makes us prone to emotional suffering. Are the personality traits that attract us to the field, ones that value order, planning, and diligence, a mismatch for the chaotic nature of human illness we treat? Or maybe there is something still flawed with medical education itself, the way it teaches us to view illness as a series of body parts and organ systems, the contradictions it forces us to navigate as we are expected to provide the best medical care to the public at what too often feels like the expense of our own well-being. Dr. Elton, and others, argue for this latter point.

In retrospect, I wonder how much these elements were at work in Cara's psychological collapse, and in my own emotional ordeal, which, ultimately, was transient. Perhaps the reforms Dr. Zaas described to me are the beginning of something sustainable. Or even transformative.

"We still have a long way to go," Dr. Zaas ultimately conceded. "Stigma remains a problem, and we need more treatment resources. But there is definitely an improved culture around seeking help. It is built into our structures now, and that's a great thing."

THE FINAL MONTHS OF INTERNSHIP YEAR BROUGHT A RETURN TO form for me. Despite the intense nature of treating patients with heart disease, lung transplants, and aggressive cancers, I remained focused and effective. Still, I increasingly looked forward to psychiatry. My medical school experience at the state hospital notwithstanding, I had since come to believe that the field held the promise of being more humane than what I would encounter if I continued on the path toward cardiology. I wanted to connect more with patients as people than merely as diagnoses, and my encounter with the social worker seemed to exemplify how that could work at its best: I'd come to his office in distress and left feeling hopeful. Certainly, many other doctors across different specialties could offer similar results, but the comparatively slower pace of psychiatry, the ability to spend more time with each person, felt like the perfect antidote to the hectic nature of hospital-based general medicine.

The more I engaged emotionally with patients, however, the more apparent it became that the marginalization of mental health concerns within medicine had clear detrimental effects on their physical and psychological well-being too, even more so than on us doctors. But not until I started working as a psychiatry resident did I begin to recognize the full extent of this harm.

PART II

FAILING PATIENTS

4

SEPARATE AND UNEQUAL

MY HANDS SQUEEZED THE STACK OF PAPERS. WAS I DOING THE RIGHT thing? Did I have a choice? I'd just handwritten a paragraph on a legal document attesting that a woman I'd interviewed a half hour earlier was a danger to herself and required involuntary hospitalization. Stephanie was in her early twenties, a part-time student and part-time waitress. She'd never been in a place like this before, literally or figuratively.

But in a span of just a few months, her life as she'd known it had fallen apart. She'd lost three people she loved. For a time, she thought she was surviving—until earlier that day, when grief and hopelessness enveloped her. She opened a bottle of ibuprofen and swallowed a handful of pills. Then within minutes, she panicked and called 911. These two acts, the overdose and then the call, brought her to my doorstep in the psychiatric emergency wing.

There, as a doctor who'd sworn to "do no harm" to patients under my care, I was about to respond to Stephanie's cry for help by sending her to the same state hospital that had distressed me so badly during medical school. Worse, the involuntary commitment papers that I held meant I'd be sending her off in handcuffs in a police car. I wouldn't know this until many years later, but it wasn't like this everywhere: in other parts of the country, state legislators took a different approach, and Stephanie would have been transported by ambulance. In that moment, though, I was acting in the only way that I knew, working within the constraints of a problematic system, and I feared Stephanie would be all the worse for it.

By then, about six months into my psychiatry residency, I'd carried out this procedure at least a dozen times without much thought. Yet as I looked at these documents, my vision went in and out of focus, my brain rattling to make sense of my actions. This process seemed not just unnecessary but possibly harmful, the opposite of serving patients. Many things in medicine involve the risk of short-term harm to meet a longer-term goal of helping someone, but this felt different. There was no option to remove a cancer-laden colon without making an incision and inserting surgical tools into the body, yet it felt like there had to be better ways to treat a depressed, recently suicidal woman than to involve law enforcement.

I had already filled in the necessary boxes on the first form and then done essentially the same thing on a second. I approached the notary on the other side of the emergency department, carrying papers that held tremendous power over Stephanie's immediate future. Then I signed the forms and the notary checked off some boxes, added her signature, and stamped the papers with a thick metal seal to make it official. My next step was to fax the pages to a magistrate office for processing. Instead, I hesitated.

I thought about the other times I'd completed this involuntary commitment process. Those patients had been experiencing acute psychosis. They were agitated, delusional, and physically threatening to others. I felt assured that we were justified to act as we did to maintain public safety. And while I had seen less severely ill patients committed, by the time I got involved, senior residents or faculty had already set the wheels in motion. Not being the primary driver of the operation in those instances had apparently kept me from considering a question that now loomed large: Why was our treatment of Stephanie being driven not by her condition alone but also by the fact that she lacked health insurance?

Stephanie had come to us voluntarily, and I was the first person from the psychiatry division to see her. In contrast to the often chronically delusional men and women who arrived at our doorstep by way of police after some public confrontation, Stephanie looked like someone who, on a better day, could be a college student preparing for final exams or a host at a nice restaurant. She spoke clearly about wanting psychiatric care, but unfortunately our inpatient unit had filled its last bed; without health insurance, no local private hospital would accept her as a transfer. And without health insurance or the ability to pay cash for private services, she had no way to get into an intensive outpatient treatment program. That left the state facility as her only option for immediate care, and signing the papers for involuntary commitment was the only way I could "help" her get there. There would be no medical gurneys or ambulance sirens; Stephanie would make the twenty-mile ride in the back of a police vehicle, handcuffed.

I held my breath and pressed Send, wincing as the machine beeped. A more humane world, one that thought differently about both health insurance and psychiatric treatment, would not have tied my hands. It would not have consigned Stephanie to what felt like a criminal proceeding on one of the worst days of her life.

DURING MY GENERAL MEDICINE INTERNSHIP, I SAW SEVERAL PAtients reject medical treatments that our team recommended. The man with uncontrolled diabetes refusing to start insulin, the woman with kidney disease and chest pain requesting to return to her apartment rather than stay overnight for observation, and so on. Unless they were badly disoriented or had no understanding of their illness and its various treatment options, we never considered forcing medical care upon them. Nor did we keep them confined to the hospital while we tried to change their minds. In these settings, most patients were allowed to make decisions about their health care, even if we felt that the interventions they refused were medically necessary and that they could suffer harm without them.

Psychiatry, in contrast, has long operated under a different set of treatment standards. Throughout nineteenth-century America, as psychiatric hospitals grew in number, and continuing into the first half of the twentieth century, when psychiatric hospitalizations peaked with over five hundred thousand beds, patients with mental illness were regarded by the general public as lacking the capability to make decisions for themselves. States assumed the power to act on behalf of these individuals' own best interests (parens patriae) and also to protect the interests of its citizens (police power); there was no distinction during this era between voluntary and involuntary hospitalizations: they all fell into the latter category.

These traditions faced intense scrutiny and backlash during the chronologically overlapping civil rights and psychiatric hospital deinstitutionalization movements of the 1950s and 1960s, and have placed increased restrictions on the ability of doctors to involuntarily hospitalize people for extended periods in our current times. Yet, as a practical matter, psychiatry is the main field of medicine where someone may understand what treatment is being offered and still be denied the right to refuse that care.

I knew none of this history when I switched from general medicine to psychiatry, and had little awareness of the ethical dilemmas that could arise with involuntary treatment. Many of the patients I'd seen to that point during my early months in psychiatry residency were diagnosed with schizophrenia or severe bipolar illness and arrived at the hospital in the throes of psychosis or mania, mental states where they often seemed genuinely dangerous to themselves or to others. On closer inspection, though, some appeared as if they might function adequately outside the hospital if better treatment structures and support systems were in place. But helping patients access those services seemed more in the realm of "social work" than "medicine." Besides, my overriding goal as new psychiatry trainee was to gain the respect of my supervisors. Who was I to question any of what was taking place around me?

Throughout the night that I met Stephanie, these contrasts between psychiatry and general medicine played in my mind. An hour before meeting Stephanie, I spoke with Ashley, another young woman who came to the ER with a similar story: an overdose triggered by various disruptions in her life. She had health insurance though, and had taken the last available bed on our small psychiatric unit. The result of these differences was stark. No police. No handcuffs. Just a friendly nurse to escort her to the upstairs unit. I'd never seen any discrepancy like that while working in general medicine. If health care could be that different for the same problem, then something indeed was wrong.

Both women had come to the hospital after 911 calls, the same way many of the patients with chest pain, bloody urine, and stroke symptoms on the medical wing presented for treatment. The fact that one woman could take the last bed on an undersized psychiatric ward, while the other woman was ushered to a state facility by police, illustrated how psychiatry, while ostensibly a mainstream medical specialty, operated at the margins.

IT WAS JUST AFTER MIDNIGHT ON A HECTIC SHIFT IN THE EMERgency department when I met Stephanie. I'd been working the 8:00 P.M. to 8:00 A.M. slot for two weeks and was looking forward to resuming a daytime schedule. Being up all night, five nights each week, had given me an appreciation, for the first time, of the sacrifices my dad made when I was growing up, as he worked nights in the frigid meat department of an inner-city grocery store. Many times, I questioned why he couldn't take me to a basketball practice or why he fell asleep for long stretches on the weekends. Now I understood.

I pushed away these childhood memories as the office phone rang.

"Hi," a woman's voice said to me through the receiver. "This is Dr. Jennings again. We've got another one for you."

Dr. Jennings was a third-year resident in the emergency medicine program, which staffed the ER twenty-four hours a day. These doctors called my wing of the ER for people who needed a "psych disposition." The overriding goal of bringing us on board was to help determine whether a patient needed a psychiatric hospital admission or could be discharged home with an outpatient treatment plan.

"Okay," I said as I picked up a nearby pencil and scrap paper. "I'm ready."

She told me Stephanie's name followed by her medical one-liner: "She's a twenty-three-year-old woman who says she took about fifteen over-the-counter ibuprofen tablets three hours ago."

If I had heard this news about a classmate, a colleague, or even a friend of a friend, I would have made some emotional connection to the situation. Or at least I would have tried. Instead, I found myself swatting away selfish thoughts about how the steady flow of patients was going to keep me busy for the next several hours.

"Any other details?" I asked.

"Medically, she's having a little abdominal pain, but it seems fairly mild, and everything else looks stable from our end. Normal vitals and labs. She's all yours."

"Any psych history?"

"No meds or previous hospitalizations or suicide attempts. From what I gather, breaking up with her boyfriend was the trigger. It sounds like you have the bad-coping-skills circuit tonight."

Dr. Jennings had called me an hour or so earlier about Ashley, who arrived with a similar story. A volatile relationship had taken a bad turn, and she'd swallowed a handful of pills. In the two weeks I'd been working nights, I'd seen four or five similar cases. There was an aphorism in emergency psychiatry circles that women preferred pills or cutting their wrists as ways to physically hurt themselves, while men gravitated toward the more lethal options of guns, hanging, or car exhaust inhalation. So far, my limited experience had supported this.

"What's the plan for our other lady?" Dr. Jennings asked, referring to Ashley.

"She's going to be admitted upstairs," I said. "I'm doing her paperwork now."

"And the schizophrenic guy? Is he all set?"

Before Ashley, I'd seen a fortysomething man whose delusions and hallucinations had gotten much worse after he'd been switched from one antipsychotic medication to a newer one his doctor hoped would cause fewer side effects. His mother, with whom he lived, called the police when he started hurling knives into a neighbor's yard.

"Yes, he's going to the state hospital," I answered.

"He's a trip," Dr. Jennings said, laughing at some of the nonsensical things he'd told the medical team. "Psych wouldn't be half-bad if you didn't have to deal with the borderline personality types. God bless you guys for being willing to take that on."

With her comments, Dr. Jennings had drawn a moral distinction, like many people do, between "real" mental illness, such as schizophrenia, and the emotional problems that would cause someone to take a dozen pills and then immediately call 911 for help.

"Okay, I'll go see her after I finish up the paperwork on this other one," I said.

"Sounds good," Dr. Jennings said. "Hopefully, it cools off for both of us from here on."

My first six months as a psychiatry resident had been a seamless transition from general medicine training. I started off on an inpatient unit, one very different from my state hospital experience in medical school. The psychiatrists at this university unit had more general medicine training, and they made the overlap between these two fields more evident. The setup for patients differed too. This ward offered single rooms and daily doctor visits, while the state hospital required shared rooming with people in varying states of emotional distress, accompanied by less frequent doctor visits, often just three times per week.

In subtle and not-so-subtle ways, the patients at the university unit weren't the same either. They all had significant psychiatric problems— intense suicidal thoughts, mania, delusions—but they generally skewed older, female, and white. During my time on the university unit, I only saw one or two black male patients, whereas at the state hospital, they came in every day. I noticed a similar if somewhat less dramatic pattern with black women too. I figured this had something to do with who had money and who didn't, and my first few days in the emergency department—the place where most people came first before being sent to any psychiatric bed—bore that out.

Shortly after I got off the phone with Dr. Jennings, ER nursing staff brought Stephanie from the medical wing of the emergency department to the psychiatric area. I swiped my badge to open the first wooden door.

This led into a small workstation area, where a nurse sat at a desk that faced an interior locked area behind a second door. The nurse was probably late forties, her lengthy graying hair bunched into a bun at the back.

"How does she seem?" I asked her, referring to Stephanie.

Nurses are important in all medical disciplines, but I found them even more vital with my transition to psychiatry. People in acute psychiatry settings, whether severely anxious or intrusively manic, often need more reassurance and direction than patients on surgery or medicine. A large part of that duty falls to nurses. From what I witnessed, they calmed people through their words and manner, lessening the need for frequent and high-dose medications. They anticipated problems with individual patients or between patients. I rarely spoke to a patient in the hospital or ER without first checking in with the assigned nurse.

"Quiet," she said. "Very sad. She's not going to be a problem for us behavior-wise. And we're going to keep Mr. Patterson as far away from her as possible."

Mr. Patterson was the knife-throwing patient with schizophrenia waiting for the sheriff to take him to the state hospital. The nurse had moved him to one of the two seclusion rooms, unsure how he might interact with Stephanie, who sat in the common area that had been divided into six small cubicles, each with a lounge chair bolted to the floor. Ashley, the other young woman I'd just seen and planned to admit upstairs, remained on the medical wing, as her overdose was deemed more severe.

I approached Stephanie. A gray blanket covered her from the neck down, underneath which her arms hugged her folded legs. Her eyes were bloodshot, the circles underneath them noticeably browner than the rest of her face. It appeared sleep had been elusive and that she'd been doing a lot of crying.

Some patients in psychiatric hospitals and emergency rooms bombard psychiatrists during initial meetings with demands to be discharged home or requests for potent drugs to tamp their anxiety. Others experience delusions and accuse us of bizarre conspiracies. Stephanie fell into a third category: passive and seemingly helpless. She wasn't going to say anything until I did. Although I was a few years older, we were both young adults, likely part of the same generation. Yet in that moment, standing over her as I did, the gulf between us seemed cavernous. I wanted to take a seat next to her to narrow that gap, the way a doctor might in a patient room in a regular hospital or a medical office, but for security purposes, there were no movable seats.

"I know people here have already asked you about what happened tonight," I began. "And I'll need to ask you more about that too later."

She nodded, appearing resigned that she had no control of her situation. "Okay."

"But first, I want to ask: Have you ever been in a psychiatric emergency room like this or been admitted to a mental health hospital before?"

She scanned the room, then her eyes fixed on the wooden door and shatterproof plexiglass window that essentially imprisoned her. She then slowly looked up at me.

"No," she said. "I've never been in any place like this."

For a split second, I tried to imagine how unsettling it might be to be in her shoes, but I quickly let that thought pass. I had information to obtain and decisions to make.

"Have you gotten outpatient therapy or counseling, or been prescribed any medications for any kind of emotional issue?" I asked.

She shook her head again. I didn't know then how common it was for people to have their initial contact with mental health treatment occur in an emergency department. My own first interaction with a mental health provider had been less than a year earlier, when I met a clinical social worker after I'd melted down during an overnight hospital shift. As nervous as I was upon meeting him, I couldn't envision how much worse that feeling would have been had it occurred in a locked facility.

I assumed she hadn't woken up the previous morning in an otherwise normal life and decided by day's end to take an overdose of pills, so instead of focusing on that act, I tried to get a sense of what led to it. I started with the boyfriend Dr. Jennings mentioned.

"He found someone else," she said. "I just wish he would've told me directly. I don't blame him. Being around me is bad luck."

"What do you mean?"

She started crying. Less than five minutes into meeting me, a white-coated stranger, Stephanie bared her pain in search of my help. In few other jobs would this occur at all, much less be routine, as it had become for me during my medical training.

"My mom," she said, sniffling every few seconds. "She died three months ago."

She explained that her mom had a massive heart attack, and after a few days in the hospital, the doctors said she had virtually no chance of surviving off life-support machines. Still, Stephanie, like many people, felt guilty about that final decision to disconnect the ventilator. Initially, her grief reached me only on a superficial level, as I was physically drained from a series of night shifts. Emotional numbing was an occupational hazard in all medical fields; psychiatry was no exception.

I recentered on her, however, as she kept talking: "I think that, you know, what happened to my brother, it broke her heart."

She went on to recount that her brother, just a year younger, had been killed in a car accident only a few months before her mom's death, when a drunk driver crossed over the yellow line and crashed into him, killing him instantly. My stomach clenched. She'd been through so much in such a short period of time. How would I have responded if the life I'd known had caved in around me so suddenly?

We then went through the details of her overdose as I tried to get a sense of how much planning went into it, what her specific intentions were, and why, thirty minutes after taking the pills, she decided to call 911 for help. The way she explained things, it appeared she had thought about suicide off and on for weeks. She chose pills because she wanted something painless that wouldn't be too messy, but got scared when her stomach started hurting. In the psychiatric terminology I was learning at the time, her suicide attempt was low-risk (didn't involve guns, jumping off a bridge, or ingesting some caustic poison) and high-rescue (she called 911 versus being discovered by chance by a friend or family member). Overall, that put her in the least worrisome bracket. Still, looking at her mournful face and having heard her story, I was concerned.

"Now that a few hours have passed since you took the pills, what do you think about everything?" I asked.

"I made a mistake," she said, looking away. "But I don't know what I should do next."

We talked through things that could keep her grounded or that she enjoyed, "protective factors" in mental health lingo. She didn't have a whole lot. No kids. No mother. No brother or other siblings. No boyfriend or close friends. Her dad was alive but distant. She'd gone to church as a kid, but religious belief wasn't part of her life any longer. She'd already withdrawn from community college for the semester. Her job as a waitress was the closest thing to an anchor that she had in the world.

"What do you think about coming into the hospital for treatment?" I asked her.

"For how long?"

That would be up to her and the doctors on the inpatient unit, I told her, but a typical admission for a case like hers was anywhere from five to ten days.

"What about my job?" she asked.

I didn't have a good answer. I assumed a restaurant couldn't fire someone specifically for having a mental health diagnosis, but I doubted they were obligated to keep her if she missed several days.

"What if I went home and got an appointment with a psychologist?" she asked.

From everything I'd seen and heard so far during residency training, what psychiatrists seemed to fear most was releasing someone from the hospital and then having that person promptly die from suicide. Admitting patients to the hospital rather than discharging them was the safer choice, especially for someone like me, just six months into my training. A full-fledged psychiatrist, one experienced in emergency assessments and more knowledgeable about available resources, might have felt differently, however.

"I think the only way that could work," I began, "is if there was someone reliable who you could stay with while you got started with treatment. What about your father?"

"Me and him aren't close," she answered softly. "We don't really talk."

We went back and forth for a bit about her options, inpatient versus outpatient, and Stephanie agreed that I could call her dad, who she thought would still be up at this hour of the night because he worked the late-evening shift at an area prison.

He picked up on the second ring: "Who's this?" he said, in a deep, harsh voice that put me on the defensive.

"I'm . . . calling about your daughter, Stephanie," I said. "I'm a doctor. She's at the hospital in the emergency room. In the psychiatric wing."

The line went silent for a few seconds. "What's she doing there?"

I explained to him that she'd taken an overdose of pills and that she needed to begin psychiatric treatment. The decision we had to make was hospital versus outpatient care and his involvement could potentially impact our approach.

The line was silent again. "I can't get that involved," he said finally. "I got two younger kids. Teenagers. And my wife's mother is staying with us now too."

I felt my hand squeeze the phone receiver tightly as the muscles in my neck clenched. I tried to envision myself in Stephanie's situation: my dad would have driven five hours in the middle of the night to support me. I didn't know this man's story, but I couldn't imagine being a father who had no time for his young-adult child in crisis.

Rather than tell Stephanie those awful details, I told her that after thinking about her situation more, I strongly recommended her admission to the hospital. She agreed. "Yes, I definitely need some help."

My "doctor" work had been done. I'd evaluated a suicidal patient, and we'd arrived at a mutually agreed-upon treatment plan. But the hard part was only beginning.

WHEN PEOPLE COME TO THE EMERGENCY DEPARTMENT FOR PSYCHI-atric reasons, they are likely to spend a lot more time there than if presenting with general medical concerns. It's not the doctor part of the visit that causes the delay most times; rather, it's everything that comes afterward. A 2016 study revealed that psychiatric ER patients are six times more likely to be transferred to another facility compared with those arriving with nonpsychiatric conditions. There are far fewer psychiatric beds relative to those addressing general medicine and surgical conditions, as these patients are likelier to lack health insurance, and those insured disproportionately receive coverage through lower-paying Medicaid programs. Ultimately, psychiatry doesn't pay the way most other medical fields do toward a hospital's bottom line.

I knew about these realities only in sketchy terms when I transferred into psychiatry and spent several months on an inpatient unit. But night by night, shift by shift in the ER, the portrait came into focus. The most important detail, I quickly learned, above all others, was a person's health insurance status. That factor would determine what treatment options were available. In the years before passage of the Affordable Care Act, most of the local private psychiatric hospitals accepted patients with good private insurance, fewer accepted Medicare, still fewer Medicaid, and almost none accepted a person without health coverage.

I didn't know where Stephanie fell on this spectrum at first because I avoided asking about her insurance. One of the faculty doctors I'd worked with on a previous shift had recommended seeing new patients this way, to eliminate the chance for preinterview bias that might occur if you knew someone's health insurance status and, by proxy, their economic standing. But would I really conduct a different interview if they had a platinum health plan versus none at all? I wanted to believe that I'd approach everyone the same. Regardless of my actions as a doctor, however, I knew that the health system itself did care about this distinction, and sorted people as a result. Some had an invitation into the club, while others were told to keep away.

After talking with Stephanie, I left the locked area and walked down a hallway toward an administrative office. There, I approached a middle-aged woman, sitting behind a glass window, who verified insurance information on each patient checked in through the ER.

"Can I help you?" she asked.

During weekday daytime hours, the ER social workers in the psychiatric wing handled this process of insurance verification and authorization. They were the ones who called outside hospitals and asked them to accept our patients. At night, and on weekends, however, this duty fell to the psychiatry resident on duty. Nothing about these tasks felt "medical" in the way I'd been taught to evaluate and treat health conditions during my years of training. No clinical sleuthing. No heroic procedures. Just boring bureaucracy.

I asked her about Stephanie.

"No insurance is listed," the woman answered.

I grimaced. I'd hoped the restaurant job, the one she feared losing, had a health plan. In my experience, few patients that I encountered had their own individual health plans, and for those that did, the mental health benefits were sparse. And to receive Medicaid in North Carolina then required one to be either pregnant, a parent to a young child, blind, elderly, or otherwise disabled. That left a lot of people who fell through the cracks, nearly one in six adults under sixty-five at the time.

I called my assigned psychiatry supervisor, Dr. Pugh, who, like all the other psychiatrists we worked under in the emergency department, took overnight calls from home.

"Hello," he said groggily.

"I've got a patient to sign out," I said.

I always felt guilty waking up senior faculty in the middle of the night, although in time, I came to realize that taking calls from home was a lot easier than being in the hospital when there was a resident on-site to do all of the work.

With other psychiatry faculty, I would typically go through a verbal presentation where I summarized the current situation in a paragraph or two, then discussed past psychiatric history, drug use history, medical problems, and so on. In the ER setting, it usually took three to five minutes. Dr. Pugh had made it clear earlier in the night that he had no patience for that. He wanted me to summarize the case and my plan in a single sentence.

"This is a young woman who took a small overdose of ibuprofen tablets who I think needs to be admitted," I said.

He asked a few clinical questions to clarify some details. He agreed with my conclusion. I already knew what his next question would be.

"What's her insurance?"

Ashley, the other young woman who had come to us an hour before Stephanie following her own overdose, had just taken the last bed on our unit. That meant Stephanie's only hospital option was transfer to another facility. We had four or five places in a fifty-mile radius to send patients when our unit was full; based on clinical criteria, she was the sort of patient they preferred: not violent, not psychotic, not manic, not drug-consuming, and physically healthy. As far as psychiatric admissions went, she fell into the "good" category.

Everything lined up except for one glaring problem. "She's uninsured," I answered.

None of these hospitals would take a patient without health coverage. They would have been obligated, at least in theory, to care for her had she shown up at their doorstep. That was the law. But they were not required to accept her from another facility, not when she lacked the means to get them paid. I talked through the different hospitals with Dr. Pugh before he told me what to do next.

"Sounds like you need to prepare the papers for the state hospital."

I sighed. This was what I had feared. All patients transferred from the ER needed a note with clinical documentation, papers with information on clinical history, vital signs, lab tests, and the like. Medical stuff. But sending someone to a psychiatric hospital required legal forms too. We had to complete "commitment paperwork," a series of forms that empowered law enforcement officers to "take custody" of people. That was the only way to get someone to a psychiatric hospital back then. Ambulances, the usual route of hospital-to-hospital transit in other settings, lost out to the convenience and certainty of using a secure police vehicle. What if the patient changed his mind and refused transfer? What if he became violent and endangered EMS personnel and other drivers on the highways?

But Stephanie had called 911 on her own, posed no apparent threat to other people, and had been fully cooperative during her time in the ER. Giving her the "police treatment" felt cruel. I lamented her fate with my boss for the night.

"Why don't we have more psychiatric beds here?" I asked. "There should be a way to keep her in this hospital. This wouldn't happen for a gen med or surgery problem."

"I wish I could give you a good answer," Dr. Pugh said. "It's above my pay grade."

In other words, it wasn't his problem. I wondered if he would have felt the same way had he talked to Stephanie up close and seen her unfolding anguish. Or maybe he had once cared about this disparity, as I did now, but, over time, had become cynical and defeated.

I asked him if we could send Stephanie home instead.

"With what sort of follow-up plan?" he asked.

This is where her lack of health insurance kicked in again. Partial hospitalization, or intensive outpatient programs, with daily or near-daily individual and group therapy care, might have been a good compromise, but Stephanie had no chance of being accepted into one without health insurance unless she had several thousand dollars' worth of disposable income sitting in her checking account.

"If she had an outpatient psychiatrist we could call who could see her tomorrow, then that might work," he continued. "But she doesn't. And without insurance, she won't be able to get in and see someone new that soon either. I understand how this plan with the police and everything isn't ideal for someone like her. But that's all we've got unfortunately."

After two weeks in the ER, I knew well what police involvement meant. A sheriff had just arrived that evening as I finished up my interview with Stephanie about a half hour earlier. Per protocol, he was going to put Mr. Patterson, the patient with worsening schizophrenia, in handcuffs and leg shackles, place him in the back of his police vehicle, and drive him across county lines to the state hospital. These procedures certainly made Mr. Patterson seem like a criminal rather than a patient in need of medical treatment, but I didn't know much about the larger world of psychiatric care and that less coercive alternatives existed, even for someone with his level of impairment. Besides, it wasn't as if I, as a new psychiatry resident, could change state, county, or hospital policies.

Even back then, though, this custodial approach felt wrong for Stephanie. She just lacked health insurance. I was desperate to come up with another plan.

MANY PEOPLE REASONABLY DREAD THE THOUGHT OF PSYCHIATRIC hospitalization, the fear of being locked away for an undetermined period of time in a place with others whose minds are equally troubled, or even more so. But there are ways that the referring facility—usually an emergency department—can ease this uncertainty before one enters a psych unit. Conversely, they can make it a lot worse. Immediately after I got off the phone with my supervisor, I saw both extremes play out as I checked in with Ashley and then Stephanie.

Ashley had come to the hospital shortly before Stephanie. Her primary care doctor had diagnosed her with depression and panic disorder a year earlier and started her on an antidepressant drug and a benzodiazepine pill to treat her symptoms. This seemed to work well initially, but less so as she started her senior year of college and became increasingly distressed about her next steps. Then, in quick succession, her father was diagnosed with colon cancer and she discovered that her boyfriend of two years had reconnected with his high school sweetheart. Several hours before I met her, she went into her bathroom and swallowed a handful of her prescription pills, which she had taken erratically the previous few weeks. Her roommate came home and found her asleep on the bathroom floor and called 911.

The emergency medicine doctors called me to see her following their clinical evaluation. Unlike Stephanie, Ashley had not been taken back to the psychiatric holding area; instead, she was in the same type of treatment room as if she'd come in with appendicitis or a kidney stone. Her overdose was deemed more medically serious.

After I talked with her for twenty minutes, Ashley and I agreed that hospital admission should be the next step, since she did not already have an outpatient therapist, and her situation was too acute for her primary care doctor to manage. Her mom, who sat at her bedside for part of my interview, felt the same. Ashley had private health insurance through her parents—her mom was an oncology nurse and her dad a pharmacist—and a bed was available for her upstairs. All I had to do was complete my physician notes and hospital orders. An ER nurse would call a psych floor nurse, and the process would unfold. Smooth and easy.

Once I'd finished speaking with Dr. Pugh about Stephanie's case, I approached Ashley's room for a final check-in before she headed upstairs. A nursing assistant sat in a tall chair right outside the entrance, her presence a "one-to-one" precaution ordered for all patients deemed a suicide or other safety risk.

"Everything okay?" I asked as I peeked inside, where Ashley looked asleep.

The woman nodded. "She just closed her eyes a few minutes ago after her mom left."

Just as I was about to knock on the sliding glass door, I heard a different female voice, one with a familiar Southern accent, call my name. I turned toward the speaker. It was a nurse from the psych unit I'd worked with months earlier. She had been gracious in helping me adjust to the differences in nursing duties between general medicine and psychiatry.

"How's our lady?" she asked me. "I'm here to bring her upstairs."

"I was just about to check in on her," I answered. "Wanna join me?"

We knocked on the door and entered once Ashley opened her eyes and saw us. With her reddish hair, freckled face, and small frame curled up under the covers on her hospital bed, Ashley looked more like a sick child than a college student on the cusp of graduation. I introduced the nurse and turned things over to her.

"Hello," she said. "I'm going to bring you upstairs and help you get settled."

She then answered several practical questions. She told Ashley where her personal belongings would be stored, when she could have visitors, and so on.

"What's it like up there?" Ashley asked. "What floor is it on?"

The nurse and I exchanged a quick glance. While it was a dramatic upgrade over the state hospital environment, our unit still had a "second-class feel" compared with other parts of the hospital. Most noticeably, it was in a different building: general medicine, neurology, surgery, pediatrics, obstetrics, oncology, cardiology, and radiology were all in the newer hospital complex, while psychiatry was left behind in the space built decades earlier. I didn't know the official explanation, but I assumed the separation was a combination of finances and stigma: psychiatric patients brought less money to the hospital, and most people not connected to the psych ward probably breathed a little easier knowing that its patients and their problems weren't too close.

We answered Ashley's question without sharing any of these concerns. The nurse reassured Ashley that she would usher her through her admission process and that the team on the unit looked forward to helping her. Ashley was in good hands. I excused myself and told her that I wished her well.

"Thanks, Doctor," Ashley replied.

"Good to see you again," the nurse said to me, smiling.

I left feeling satisfied. Yes, Ashley's situation was clearly unenviable: She'd decided just hours earlier to overdose and was headed to a locked ward, a place she'd never been before. Her future was uncertain. But her transition from ER doctor, to me, to the nurse transporting her to the unit had been seamless. We'd made the best of bad circumstances.

My optimism faded as I dragged myself over to the psychiatric wing to speak with Stephanie. She was the only patient in the locked unit at that point, the man with schizophrenia having been shipped to the state hospital. But the nursing assistant looked as if she was preparing to bring another patient back.

"Someone else coming?" I asked the psychiatric nurse.

"Man with bipolar who is manic," she said. "Might have another on the way too."

I closed my eyes briefly. Patients were coming one after the other. I felt a sudden urgency to sort out Stephanie's situation quickly. She looked up as I approached.

"I talked with my psychiatry supervisor and the senior ER doctor on duty," I began, "and they agree on your being admitted to the hospital for further care."

"Okay," she said. "When will that happen? Which floor will I be on?"

If she had come in with bloody diarrhea or an infected gallbladder, she certainly would have been transported to a medical or surgical floor within the hospital. But with the physical effects of her overdose being relatively mild, her issue was deemed "psychiatric," and that made for an entirely different bed-availability situation.

"We don't have any available beds here," I said.

She frowned. "So what does that mean?"

I looked down at my folded hands, then back up at her. "Our plan is to transfer you to the state hospital," I said.

"Where is that?"

"About twenty miles away."

Stephanie stared back, accepting. Clearly, the "state hospital" didn't mean anything more to her than it had to me before I rotated there as a medical student. It was a world most "normal" people didn't have to think about. I felt like I had to begin to prepare her.

"The main thing about that," I said, "is that you won't go there by ambulance, like you came here. Instead, the police will have to take you there."

Stephanie put her face into her hands. "The police? But I didn't do anything . . ."

No, she hadn't done anything wrong in a legal sense, as she rightly protested. But had she died from suicide, we would have all said at the time that she'd "committed" suicide, the same language people use when someone perpetrates robbery, treason, rape, or manslaughter. Society, and medicine, then and now, had a long way to travel before it could view suicide as being closer to a stroke than to a sin. Maybe that wasn't fully possible.

"Can I just go home?" she asked.

Discharging her home in the middle of the night, just a few hours after an overdose, back to her apartment alone, without any family support or, more important, the ability to schedule an appointment? Dr. Pugh already said he wasn't going to sign off on that. But I did have another idea, a last-ditch effort.

"Let me check on something," I said. "I'll be back in a few minutes."

I left the locked wing and trotted to the medical wing workstations, where I found Dr. Jennings, the resident I'd talked with earlier, and her supervisor, a late-fiftyish guy who seemed a little too old for the night shift. I asked them if we could keep Stephanie in the holding area overnight, until she could be reevaluated in the morning.

"What would that change?" he asked.

Maybe Stephanie might think of a responsible friend or extended family member we could contact during normal hours, I told him. Or our psychiatric unit would get an unexpected discharge and a bed would open up for her.

The two doctors exchanged a brief, questioning glance before the supervisor spoke.

"This patient has a reasonable plan in place," he said, referring to the state hospital. "I hear your concerns in her case, but there is no way we can justify keeping her here another seven or eight hours on the small chance that we might be able to come up with something different in the morning or afternoon. I wish I could give you different news."

ERs are tracked on how quickly they see patients and how long it takes for them to be sent either up (hospital admission) or out (discharge or transfer). They must be ready for the next . . . emergency. In that sense, Stephanie needed to be moved along to make room for the next case. That was what the health care system demanded.

Suddenly, another Hail Mary came to me.

"The patient we're admitting to psych," I began, referring to Ashley, speaking fast as I tended to when I felt unsettled. "Can't we just send her to a medicine floor? Her overdose was more serious. That way we could admit the other woman to our psychiatric unit instead of sending her to the state hospital."

The senior ER doctor exchanged a smile with his junior doctor. "I really admire your persistence and advocacy," he told me, his expression sincere. "I used to be that way too. But for this situation, the administrative wheels have been set in motion."

He told me that we would have to discharge Ashley from the psychiatric unit and then have her come back to the emergency room and start the entire process over again, all so we could play musical beds when, in their minds, there existed a perfectly reasonable plan. No one in what was called *hospital bed control* was going to allow that to happen.

I was out of options. It was time to get the paperwork started for Stephanie's transfer to the state hospital.

Stephanie cried again as I shared this news. She told me that police made her uneasy, especially after an uncle was injured during a traffic stop. I told her that, by policy, the officer who would end up transporting her would be a woman and that we would talk to that person to explain the situation as best we could. That was all we could do. But I knew that the officer would ultimately handcuff Stephanie in transit, the way they did all of their state hospital transports. She would follow procedure, the same way the doctors had.

I spent the next several minutes completing Stephanie's paperwork, medical first, then the legal documents needed to transfer her to the state hospital. After I'd finished, I checked in with the nurse in the psychiatric wing to update her.

"This whole thing doesn't make sense," I said to her. "She comes to the hospital willingly, but we have to end up committing her."

"It's just the way it is," the nurse answered, her defeated perspective in line with the ER doctor and my psychiatry supervisor. "As good a job as they do on the other side with medical and surgical emergencies, with psych, things just aren't set up to make it work the best for our patients. We're an afterthought."

I wanted to keep fighting for Stephanie. But I couldn't override the decisions the ER supervisor and the psychiatrist on call had advised. And even if I could have somehow miraculously persuaded them to reconsider, it sounded like the people above them would have vetoed any change of plans. Besides, I was tired and had to start thinking about my-self. It was almost two o'clock in the morning, and my shift wasn't quite halfway done. I'd been seeing patients back-to-back the entire time, and another new one had just arrived.

I INITIALLY DIDN'T SEE STEPHANIE'S CASE THROUGH A RACIAL LENS, busy as I was navigating being the overnight in-house psychiatrist. But during a short break later that shift, I began to make those connections. The difference between what Ashley experienced—nurse escort to the university psych floor—and Stephanie being taken in police handcuffs to the state hospital was so glaring it could have been written in some textbook attempting to demonstrate what racism looked like. Only the people involved in the process, as the saying goes, "didn't have a racist bone in their bodies," as best I could tell.

Certainly, as the primary doctor on both cases, I didn't want things to play out as they did. Nor, it seemed, did other doctors do anything to put their thumb on a racial scale. Dr. Jennings, the emergency medicine resident, had dismissed both women as "emotionally fragile" while her supervisor seemed to genuinely empathize with my predicament. Dr. Pugh—the psychiatrist I'd spoken with on the phone—didn't know their racial identities; I had deliberately left out those details, as I gen-erally preferred to do. No one in our emergency department had set out in advance to privilege Ashley and harm Stephanie. If there was indeed racism, it had happened without any individual racists.

But even if Stephanie's ordeal wasn't explicitly racist, it certainly felt like part of a larger history of such mistreatment, a potent mixture of racist actions and racist inactions. In the slavery era, prominent phy-sician Samuel Cartwright put forth the diagnosis of drapetomania, the theory that only mental illness would prompt slaves to flee their captors. Early-twentieth-century psychiatrists frequently asserted that black people lacked the intelligence to benefit from psychotherapy. Schizophrenia diagnoses skyrocketed among black men during the civil rights era (after all, why else would they be so angry?), and with it, ongoing justification for more coercive treatment. In more recent times, black people are about 50 percent less likely to receive treatment for outpatient mental health problems yet are two to three times more likely to be involuntarily committed to a hospital, as Stephanie was. Given this historical legacy, it is little wonder that the relationship of black Americans to the mental health field has so often been rooted in aversion and skepticism.

While general medicine and surgical fields have their own lengthy track records of harmful bias, the particulars of where psychiatry sits within medicine makes these class-based distinctions (which so often overlap with race) starker. Not once during my medical internship year did the conversation about a patient's health coverage dominate at the outset. If someone came to the emergency department with chest pain that was determined to have a life-threatening cause, they were going to be hospitalized upstairs, not sent elsewhere. That said, a patient's health insurance status could definitely impact discharge planning—what type of rehab facility they could be sent to, the quality of their outpatient aftercare, and so on. But the initial decision of whether to admit, to not admit, or to transfer elsewhere was not so nakedly rooted in whether one had a good health plan.

Psychiatry beds, in contrast to medical and surgical beds, essentially operate under a separate system of funding from health insurance organizations and government budgets—one with considerably less revenue. Hospitals respond to this in predictable ways. Between 2005 and 2010 alone, the total number of psychiatric beds in the US decreased by 14 percent. And even patients who can find a bed may not be able to afford the help. Private mental health hospitals can cost more than $30,000 a month, and many do not accept insurance—at least not public insurance (Medicare or Medicaid). What is then left, for Stephanie and others like her, are local mental health systems that have been victim to budget cuts and the resulting shortage of available care that ensues.

With each passing day, I was coming face-to-face with the sobering reality that psychiatry was separate and on unequal footing compared with the rest of medicine. And that these class-based distinctions, for predictable historical reasons, all too often played out along racial lines. Stephanie got clobbered by both forces.

HOW MIGHT STEPHANIE'S CASE HAVE TURNED OUT DIFFERENTLY had she shown up today, more than fifteen years later? To help me try to make sense of that question, I spoke with several of my colleagues and supervisors at Duke and the Durham VA health systems. What struck me immediately was how different my experience in residency training had been from many of those who had trained in other states.

"We rarely did the police or handcuff thing," one psychiatrist told me, who'd trained in a northern state. "Only if the patient had a history of violence or was dangerously agitated and posed a true safety risk. Someone like your patient would not have been transported that way."

Instead, patients like Stephanie were shuttled by ambulance, with an attendant sitting with them, in much the same way that patients on medical floors who needed closer behavioral monitoring had sitters close at hand, similar to what Ashley had in the emergency department.

"As soon as I arrived and learned about how things worked here," my senior colleague continued, "I was so shocked and upset."

The policy extended far beyond the hospital where I trained. By law, in North Carolina, sheriffs' deputies were the default transportation means from one hospital to another for psychiatric admissions. The contrast between Stephanie's experience and what it might have been like in another state prompted me to contact Dr. Dinah Miller, a Baltimore-area psychiatrist affiliated with the Johns Hopkins University School of Medicine and prolific author on psychiatric issues. In 2016, Miller, along with psychiatrist colleague Dr. Annette Hanson, published the book *Committed: The Battle over Involuntary Psychiatric Care*, a comprehensive yet highly readable exploration of this subject.

"A discussion of involuntary care in this country is really fifty-one discussions," she told me, referencing each US state plus Washington, DC. "What's true for North Carolina isn't necessarily the case for your neighbors in Virginia or South Carolina."

Her statement, undoubtedly true, perplexed me. Sure, there are controversial issues that can intersect with medical practice (abortion, medical marijuana, transgender care, and physician-assisted suicide, to name a few) resulting in treatment options with widely different availability across America. But I couldn't understand why there were such disparate state-by-state approaches to how we evaluated and triaged mental health crises in the emergency department. Did psychiatric care, at its core, share similar moral, religious, and, ultimately, political tensions?

Unlike these other contentious areas, though, there seems to be an evolving consensus, even on a national level, that treating mental illness is a bipartisan issue. Locally, North Carolina legislators passed a law that went into effect in 2019 that enabled counties to consider alternatives to law enforcement officers transporting patients. UNC and Duke, two of the largest North Carolina health facilities, are both in the early stages of implementing a different approach to the decades-long status quo. More recently, in early 2023, North Carolina became the fortieth state to expand Medicaid under the Affordable Care Act, extending health coverage to an estimated six hundred thousand residents. People like Stephanie will now have more affordable options to receive general medical and mental health care.

While we await those changes, other reforms exist now that could have made a dramatic difference for Stephanie then.

"We actually have a full team who staffs the psych emergency room," one of Duke's psychiatry department leaders told me. "It is so different from when you were a resident."

Indeed, a complement of social workers, physician assistants, nurse practitioners, and psychiatrists allows for more detailed assessments and treatment planning than one overworked, inexperienced psychiatry trainee, as I was then, could possibly offer. Instead of the rush to send her to the state hospital, the emergency medicine doctors might have agreed to have Stephanie stay until the daytime shift arrived. Upon seeing her, this team could have decided that it made more sense to keep her in the ER until a bed became available upstairs, or with their additional experience, they may have had connections to local treatment resources and come up with a sound plan for discharge.

As our conversation continued, I found myself imagining Stephanie receiving this idealized emergency care in our almost-brand-new mental health facility. I became enthralled by the idea that, through the power of this conversation and my own thinking, I could somehow rewrite the past. But shortly after the Zoom meeting ended, my mind snapped back to visualize the reality of what actually occurred.

WHEN THE FEMALE POLICE OFFICER ARRIVED TO TRANSPORT STEPH-anie, I was seeing the next patient, a thirtyish guy with manic symptoms, convinced that he had divine powers and that his coworkers, the police, and his doctors were all his persecutors. I stepped away long enough to join the nurse in speaking with the officer. We told her our concerns with sending Stephanie to the state hospital, essentially as a prisoner, but that we had no other options. The officer, a black woman, seemed pleasant and understanding, but told us that, like us, she couldn't deviate from protocol: Stephanie would have to be handcuffed. We accepted her explanation, although that didn't make it go down any easier. I didn't watch as she took Stephanie away.

The rest of the shift stayed busy. The patient with mania was followed by a call upstairs from the main hospital: an elderly man on the surgical floor had become agitated, and they needed to know what medication to give to calm him overnight. Soon after that, another patient arrived for me to see, this one seeking treatment for his alcohol and cocaine use. Being preoccupied in this way was probably best, as it distracted me from thinking about Stephanie and the role that I had played in what took place.

In the ensuing weeks, there would be other suicide attempts and involuntary commitments, but nothing like Stephanie. She had come to us in desperation, and although we had prevented her from killing herself in the short term, it all felt so punitive. Would she ever seek mental health treatment again? Might it have been possible that, in the end, we had done more harm than good?

Of course, things may have turned out well for Stephanie. At the state hospital, she might have come to recognize that her life was indeed precious and that no matter the hardships she'd faced, she had something positive to offer this world. Maybe she got linked to an outpatient therapist or was prescribed a medication, or some combination, that helped further lift her spirits. I'd never know.

What I did know, even then, was that there had to have been a better way to manage her crisis, one that did not put her in handcuffs. More psychiatric beds to reduce the need for hospital transfers from emergency departments. Dedicated public funding to support private hospitals in accepting uninsured patients. Specialized ambulance services that could cater to a mental health clientele. And so forth.

If only more people understood her plight, I told myself that night and the ones that followed, society would deliver a better solution. As a brand-new psychiatrist in training, working under the direction of more senior doctors (themselves part of a vast, complex health care system that interfaced with an even bigger government universe), I could only hope.

5

ON PILLS AND NEEDLES

"THAT'S A LOAD OF BULLSHIT!" CRAIG BURST OUT FURIOUSLY. "ARE you really telling me that's the best we can do? She deserves a whole lot more than that."

As one of the lead nurses in the emergency department, Craig had a reputation among residents for inserting himself into doctors' treatment decisions. It had never bothered me beforehand; I took it as a sign that he cared about the patients we saw. But on this day, his words unnerved me. He'd never gone this far in challenging one of us, not that I'd seen or heard. And what he said was absolutely true.

I had just informed him that Natalie, a young woman who had terrible experiences while deployed to Iraq, could not be admitted to the hospital unit upstairs. In the years following her discharge from the army, she started consuming opioids: over time, in greater quantity and by more dangerous means. A few hours earlier, she reached a low point, a threshold she vowed never to cross, and came to our hospital begging for help. Yet instead of a safe haven within our hospital walls, or somewhere similar, we planned to send her home with papers telling her that she'd get a phone call in a few days.

"We can't admit someone strictly for opioid withdrawal," I stammered.

"But we admit addicts all the time," Craig fired back.

Indeed, people with substance-related woes came to our emergency room often. Earlier in my shift, I admitted George, a fiftysomething guy who'd been drinking about a fifth of liquor daily for several months. More alcohol each day than I consumed in an entire year.

"Opioid withdrawal isn't life-threatening like alcohol withdrawal is," I said.

My education in addiction medicine up to that point—a lecture or two during medical school and the same so far in residency training— instructed me that withdrawing from opioids, while agonizing for many, was not a life-or-death medical emergency. The way they'd taught me, substitute drugs like methadone and buprenorphine were reserved for specialized outpatient treatment settings. Nothing about opioid with-drawal required treating it in the hospital on its own, unless, for exam-ple, the person needed IV antibiotics for a serious infection related to using contaminated needles. Before this night, I'd never had occasion to question any of what I'd been told.

In contrast to opioids, I'd learned that alcohol withdrawal, in severe cases, could result in seizures, delirium, and possibly even death. The man I'd admitted earlier that evening had, during a previous admission the year before, required a week's stay in the intensive care unit to med-ically detoxify from alcohol.

Craig wasn't impressed by my medical explanation. "So we keep tak-ing in the drunks? What good does that do anybody if we know they're going to go right back to it?"

"He has a point," said Rebecca, the nurse who'd worked most closely with Natalie. "That guy who went up a few hours ago, this is his ninth admission in the last two years."

"Maybe we should have come up with a plan to send him home in-stead," Craig said.

I could have gotten defensive, as some doctors did when their judg-ment was questioned. But a part of me agreed with him. In my short time at this Veterans Affairs (VA) hospital, I'd seen a lot of middle-aged men with long histories of cycling in and out of various hospitals for al-cohol detoxification. Revolving care that sometimes made the work feel pointless. Yet I hadn't given much thought to how using resources in this way might restrict their availability in other instances. What Craig said next, though, made sense to me, especially because of how it connected to what I'd learned about chronic medical diseases.

"This girl has never reached out for help," he continued. "This is her first time. Now is the chance for us to maybe make a difference."

In my medical training so far, professors had talked often about the importance of early intervention for chronic disease like diabetes, rheumatoid arthritis, and glaucoma. Even with new drugs and other treatments constantly in development, the ideal outcome of a cure or outright prevention was often not possible. So detection and management at the earliest stages was the next-best thing. By that logic, Craig's point seemed valid; it made sense that a young person less than a year into their drug problem stood a better chance of success with the right treatment than someone who had misused alcohol for decades.

Feeling less confident by the minute, I tried to explain how the outpatient clinic—a place I'd never seen—could meet Natalie's needs. Craig wasn't persuaded.

"What about all those crack addicts we admit?" he fired back. "No one dies from coming off crack."

It was true that cocaine withdrawal didn't typically cause life-threatening medical symptoms like alcohol did. But as a stimulant drug, withdrawal often triggered severe depression in people who used it heavily. In the ER, we saw many patients in that state. Some described being suicidal. And on that basis, they were admitted to our hospital.

"And a lot of them are exaggerating," Rebecca said. "Three hots and a cot."

I bristled, since the patients who came to our ER for crack-related issues skewed black, and doctors and nurses alike often assumed, pejoratively, that they were just looking for a warm meal and a place to sleep on the government's dime. I sometimes found myself thinking that way too, but hearing these two white nurses—both of whom had always been nice to me—activated my racial reflexes. But as a very tall black man, I'd been conditioned over time not to come across as too "aggressive" or "threatening."

"They probably come to the hospital," I said calmly, "because of how bad things are on the outside."

"Sure," Craig conceded. "But that's not our responsibility to fix social problems."

Our exchange made me consider how Natalie differed from the typical patient we saw beyond the particulars of the drug that she used. Yes, Natalie was white, and even then, I was well aware of the sentencing disparity that existed between possessing powder cocaine, more commonly used by white people, and crack cocaine, whose consumers, due to cost considerations among other factors, leaned black. But the contrasts didn't stop there. Natalie was half the age of the typical veteran we saw for drug-related concerns. Youth, in many people's eyes, meant a life that held greater value. Finally, being a woman, especially given what she faced, made Natalie seem more vulnerable, needing protection in a way a belligerent drinker did not. I wondered how important these factors were in how Craig and Rebecca viewed Natalie compared to George, our older, black, repeat, repeat, repeat customer. And how much were these contrasts playing out, subconsciously, in my own mind?

"Is there some other way you could keep her?" asked Rebecca. "I mean, she clearly has PTSD."

Most of the patients we saw in the psychiatric emergency setting at the VA hospital, in fact, did not have serious substance-related problems. At least not as their only concern. Post-traumatic stress disorder (or PTSD, as it's better known) dominated our caseload. Often, these men were veterans of the Vietnam War. When I saw Natalie, however, we were beginning to get veterans from the post-9/11 Iraq and Afghanistan conflicts. And as I was learning, more of them were women. This factor brought additional considerations.

"Yes, it definitely seems that she has PTSD," I agreed. "But she's not suicidal, and what she wants is treatment for opioids, which is not considered a medical emergency."

Rebecca frowned. "The two are connected. That doesn't really make any sense."

I agreed. I felt terrible about what I was saying, but I didn't have any power to change rules. "I'll ask my supervisor," I said, "but I'm pretty sure he's going to say that we can't admit her for a primary opioid problem. Besides, we only have one bed left, and I'm sure he wants to keep it available for the usual sort of cases we admit."

Craig looked at me, resigned. "Well, that stinks, Doc, doesn't it?"

My stomach and mind both unsettled, I left the ER and headed to a secluded workstation area to phone my attending supervisor. By the time I'd dialed his number, I'd stopped thinking about Craig and started focusing on the person who really mattered here, Natalie. She'd been through so much, and despite my preaching about following the rules, I realized how strongly I'd started hoping I could find a way to help get her life on a better track. I didn't know it then, but her story was soon to be a familiar one throughout America, part of what later came to be known as the opioid epidemic.

BEFORE MEDICAL SCHOOL, I DIDN'T THINK MUCH ABOUT PAIN OR pain medications. I'd had a few basketball injuries in high school and college, but none that required more than a few days of over-the-counter pills. The same was true for my mom, whose knees and shoulders occasionally had a flare-up. On the rare occasion I thought about opioids, the image that came to mind was of a homeless person injecting heroin in an inner-city alley. That was the prejudiced assumption that pervaded news reports and scripted television back then. But unknown to me, and many others, opioids were beginning to assume a much more prominent role within the medical world and in the national consciousness.

The epidemic traces its origins to two events in 1996, coincidentally the year that I started medical school. At the annual meeting of the American Pain Society, the keynote speaker made what seemed at the time a radical proposal: "If pain were assessed with the same zeal as other vital signs are," he said, "it would have a much better chance of being treated properly. We need to train doctors and nurses to treat pain as a vital sign."

Soon thereafter, influential national health organizations and accrediting agencies adopted the slogan of pain as the "fifth vital sign" alongside the long-standing vital measurements of body temperature, pulse, blood pressure, and respiratory rate. Doctors and nurses began routinely screening people on a numeric rating scale (0–10), and patients now had more opportunity to describe their concerns. With increasing identification came more doctor interventions, and patients with low back pain and other non-cancer-related pain started getting prescriptions with greater frequency. After years of marginalization, pain—acknowledging it, measuring it, and treating it—had gone mainstream. On one hand, this represented true progress; but in this case, the timing torpedoed its good intentions.

Coinciding with this more aggressive assessment and treatment of pain was a new drug that soon reached blockbuster status. OxyContin, a longer-acting version of oxycodone from Purdue Pharma, entered the market in 1996 and within a few years became a billion-dollar drug. Part of its appeal was rooted in the perception, widely cultivated by its representatives and later proven to be false, that the long-acting properties of OxyContin significantly lowered the risk for addiction.

But even as opioids became more acceptable in medical practice, they did so in an environment where drug use itself remained highly stigmatized. During my medical internship year, our team admitted a woman in her forties with a history of high blood pressure following an episode of stroke-like symptoms, termed a transient ischemic attack, or TIA. We assumed that her medical problems had a clear emotional trigger: a week earlier, her teenage niece was killed in a bicycle accident. She missed several days of her blood pressure medication and slept poorly. We were all struck by the gut-wrenching description of the crash.

Because the patient had acknowledged recent marijuana use, our supervisor told us to get a urine drug screen. When the results detected not only marijuana but cocaine, our team's reaction to the patient abruptly changed.

"Well, now we know why she had a TIA," the attending said, with seeming certainty.

"I wonder what else is really going on with her," the resident responded.

I also felt deceived, that the woman had played with our sympathies. But why? Sure, cocaine use could potentially elevate blood pressure and cause stroke-like symptoms. But we had no way to know that this alone had caused her TIA. She might have snorted a single time a few days earlier, yet we instantly assumed, knowing little about her life, that this woman was a habitual drug user who'd caused her own problems. Perhaps she'd feared exactly this kind of judgment when she decided not to disclose her cocaine use to us. Or she herself was ashamed of using drugs. Still, as our emotions toward her chilled, the fact remained that her teenage niece had been killed when a driver ran a red light. How did the results of a drug test make that reality any less tragic or make this woman any less deserving of our attention?

When I switched specialties the following year, I soon saw that psychiatrists weren't necessarily more sympathetic toward patients who used drugs. A few months before I met Natalie, I was covering the walk-in mental health clinic when a man in his fifties arrived complaining of anxiety. He asked for clonazepam, a sedative he'd been given a few years before by a local physician when his wife was diagnosed with breast cancer. Her cancer had returned, and he wanted to restart it. I asked him about getting counseling, but he was focused on medication to ease his distress. Clonazepam can be addictive and is misused by some people, although others take it appropriately to help dampen their anxiety.

"I need something to take the edge off," he said. "I could drink a six-pack each day, but I assume it's safer to get a prescription to calm my nerves."

I talked to him about the SSRI class of drugs—Prozac, Zoloft, and others. He said he'd tried one of those before and didn't like how it made him feel. He also wanted something that he could take when he needed it, not a daily pill like an SSRI.

I left the room to talk with my supervisor that day, who was working in another part of the hospital. He looked at the patient's electronic record as I presented the case.

"They always have a story, don't they?" he said after I'd finished.

He then explained the challenge of treating what he termed "pill seekers," people who want a drug to fix every problem in their lives. I understood what he meant, yet was surprised at how detached he sounded.
Having a fifty-year-old wife with recurrent breast cancer seemed a lot
more overwhelming than the more mundane stresses of life that often
brought patients our way seeking help. But my supervisor was the one
with the years of experience, so I followed his lead.

"Well, he might not have been getting clonazepam for the past year,"
he continued, "but he likes drugs. His urine was positive for marijuana.
And he's a heavy smoker. From my read of his chart, he just wants pills.
I'm sure he'll go out and find some on the street when you tell him no. But
at least your name—and mine—won't be on the prescription."

His cynicism surprised me. Earlier in the shift, this same psychiatrist
had talked with great compassion about a Vietnam veteran with PTSD
and a young mom with severe depression. No moral judgment. Only
caring. Yet the specter of problematic drug use seemed to elicit an entirely different reaction. I wondered if I might become that pessimistic
in the future. Had I already started down that path without realizing it?

Even then, I observed that while many of us in psychiatry and general medicine increasingly embraced biological models of depression,
anxiety, and bipolar disorder, we often still saw alcohol and drug use
differently, a problem of an individual's own making. Our language
communicated this distaste. We described urine toxicology samples as
"dirty" or "clean," and patients with drug problems had "dysfunctional
personalities" and were commonly referred to as "abusers" or "addicts"
or "alcoholics." During clinical interviews, we sought to determine the
person's "drug of choice" that required our attention. I freely used these
terms with colleagues to describe patients without giving thought as to
how it might impact the care they received.

What was behind these disparaging words and hostile reactions?
While many of us brought some of that ill will with us into our medical
training, given the widespread societal stigma against those with drug
problems, our medical indoctrination likely worsened it.

"Doctors are trained to feel deeply responsible for fixing other people's

problems," Dr. Christine Wilder, a psychiatrist and addiction specialist at the University of Cincinnati, told me. "And then when someone
has a disease that affects their judgment such that they reject, ignore, or
mislead the physician who feels responsible for fixing them, the doctor
experiences a sense of failure."

And while few people relish the idea of failure, it is especially anath-
ema to doctors, who thrived in the premed crucible and envisioned a career saving lives or, at least, dramatically improving them.

"Feeling like you're failing is extremely uncomfortable for physicians,"
Dr. Wilder continued, "so blaming the person causing that emotion is
much easier to tolerate."

Indeed, one of the few things that seemed to unite many doctors and
nurses was a disdain for those with drug problems. Especially if these
individuals were "repeat offenders" because, in our view, their plight was
"completely self-inflicted."

As the concept of pain, and the drugs to relieve it, became increasingly acceptable topics to address in medicine, embracing the individuals whose pain led to drug misuse, and devising strategies to address
these concerns, lagged considerably behind. Natalie's case brought this
dilemma into clear view.

WHEN I GOT THE CALL FROM THE ER TO SEE NATALIE, I MOMENTAR-
ily thought I was at the wrong hospital. It was 4:00 A.M., and the shriek
of my pager startled me from deep slumber. The nurse, Rebecca, started
off by referring to the patient as "Ms."

"You sure?" I asked, my head throbbing and my eyes blinded by the
overhead light I'd just turned on. "It's a woman?"

"I think I know the difference," she replied sarcastically. "Nurses are
smart too."

"Of course, of course," I stammered. "Sorry . . . so sorry about that.
Just waking up. I'm just not used to seeing women here."

Women comprised around half the patients at the other hospitals
I'd worked at during my training, but well below 10 percent at the VA

facility where I'd spent the last several weeks. The math was simple: despite women entering the military in greater numbers over time, the service branches remained overwhelmingly male. Most veterans we saw had been on active duty when those ratios were even further skewed toward men.

Rebecca told me our patient was twenty-six years old and requested drug detox. Midtwenties seemed young for the age of the psychiatric patients we typically saw there.

"What drugs?" I asked.

"Opioids," she replied. "We're checking her drug screen to see what else she has on board. She says the only other thing she does is smoke cigarettes on occasion. Nothing else."

The typical drug screen we used also tested for cocaine, marijuana, amphetamines, benzodiazepines, and barbiturates. Patients often took these drugs simultaneously or in close succession, and weren't always forthcoming about using them, for all sorts of reasons. Many patients also drank alcohol and smoked cigarettes. We could draw blood to measure alcohol levels. With nicotine, we really didn't give it much thought in the acute setting, unless the patient had a known lung problem; rather than lab data, we unscientifically relied on how yellow-stained their nails were.

"What are her vitals?" I asked.

"BP is a little high—138/92. Heart rate up a bit too, about 105. Her temp is normal. So are her breathing rate and O_2 sat."

Nothing life-threatening. I quickly thought through what I recalled about opioids in intoxication and withdrawal phases. Too much could cause pinpoint pupils, sedation, and slowed breathing; in overdose, coma and death. Coming off could result in dilated pupils, diarrhea, cramps, sweating; nothing that would kill you, as I understood things.

"Any SI?"

SI was our shorthand for *suicidal ideation*. No suicidal thoughts, Rebecca answered.

"Anything in her chart?" I asked.

"First time here," she said. "Or any VA from what I can tell from our system."

In medical school, new cases like this brought excitement, an investigation into the unknown. By the time I was in the thick of medical internship, however, I longed for patients where the clinical history was already documented and the treatment plans were straightforward. Some of that earlier enthusiasm returned when I switched into psychiatry, but not for long; I found a certain calm working on autopilot, especially in the predawn hours of a Saturday morning when I was twenty hours into a twenty-four-hour shift.

Natalie was in the primary "psych room" at the time, a square-shaped area the size of a bedroom in a middle-income house, only without the furniture. The floors were dingy vinyl, and the bare walls felt wholly uninviting. She sat on a gurney pushed against the rear wall, her feet dangling off the bed. I sat down in a rolling chair I'd wheeled into the room, positioned such that we were basically eye level with each other.

"Hello," I said.

She glanced at me, then quickly away, then back again. A nursing aide had helped her change into paper hospital scrubs. The unforgiving fluorescent lighting revealed clues about her recent emotional state. She had dark spots underneath her bloodshot eyes, set against an oily, otherwise pale complexion. Her hair needed a good wash and conditioning. My initial reaction was that life had been hard on her, probably a lot more so than most. Still, underneath the signs of despair, I tried to envision her in a happier time, before the drug problems that had brought her to the hospital. My imagination could not take me there.

"Can you keep the door open?" she asked. "Nurse Rebecca said she was going to stay with me while I talked with you."

Some patients with psychosis I'd met were afraid to be alone with me in a room, fearing that I was an enforcer of a convoluted government plot to persecute them. And on occasion, I worried about being alone with some of them, given their detachment from reality. But Natalie's plea, I suspected, had a different cause. I obliged.

"She got called to help with another patient," I told her, "but said she'd come back when she could. Is it okay if we start without her?"

"Sure," Natalie said softly.

"Why did you decide to come to the emergency room tonight?" I asked.

She grimaced as she clutched her stomach with her right hand briefly, then used the back of her left hand to wipe away sweat along her temples.

"I need help," she replied. "I have a problem."

Sometimes patients exaggerated their distress to get a doctor to take them seriously, or to get a desired treatment. But cramps and sweating were known symptoms of opioid withdrawal. I tried to keep an open mind.

"The nurse, Rebecca, told me you've been using a lot of opioids."

She nodded as she shut her eyes.

"What type?"

Opioids came in several varieties and people ingested them in different ways. Some swallowed. Some chewed. Others crushed and snorted. Still others filled a syringe and injected them through a vein.

"I started with pills. Vicodins, Percocets. Oxys. Prescription stuff."

"How long ago did that begin?"

"I hurt my knee in the army," she began, "and it never got right. I hurt it more in a car accident after I got out. A doctor at an urgent care gave me some Vicodin. That was over a year ago. Before that, I'd never been someone who drank a lot or used drugs."

"And when did you start feeling like the pills were a problem?"

"I don't know exactly. But at some point, I realized that it wasn't just about my knee. The pills helped me not feel so stressed out."

My first experience taking opioids was when a dentist prescribed a dozen to me after removing my four wisdom teeth. The pills helped numb the surgical pain those first two days, but they also made my stomach hurt. More important, I didn't feel any different from a psychological standpoint, so I was happy to throw the last few in the trash when the pain began to subside. I wondered whether the difference in our responses to these same medications was biologically determined or due to our contrasting life circumstances. How might I have responded had those pills made me feel "good" or "whole" in some way? Would I have found a way to get another prescription? Or two? Or three?

"So what led up to your coming today?" I asked. "What's happened more recently?"

Natalie started crying as she explained how one doctor who'd given her opioids found out another doctor was prescribing them too, and they both stopped at the same time. She then started buying them on the street from some high school acquaintances, but that eventually proved too costly. To satisfy her opioid need, she found something much cheaper and did something she never thought she'd do:

"I took heroin," she said as tears streamed down her face and snot from her nostrils. "Three days ago. And then the next day. And then yesterday."

"How did you ingest it?" I asked as I handed her a tissue.

She blew her nose for a good ten seconds. "I snorted it the first two days. But then yesterday I was using with this other girl, and she showed me how to inject it. My mom found out. I promised her I would stop. So I came here."

I thought about the time in high school when my mom discovered that I'd figured out a way to unscramble some adult movie station. The shame sickened me for days. I couldn't imagine what that might have felt like had she caught me using cocaine or heroin.

Natalie explained that heroin came a lot cheaper than OxyContin. My only other experiences in training with heroin users had occurred with a man with end-stage AIDS and a woman with a destroyed heart valve. Those were people whose heroin use had ravaged their bodies and whom I'd thought of in terms of their diseased organ systems rather than as individuals. I tried to square those earlier encounters with the woman in front of me, whom I was engaging with on a human level.

This was the first time I'd heard what would become a familiar story: an initial doctor's prescription leading to ongoing refills and renewals that morphed into buying pills from small-time dealers before metasta-sizing into snorting, smoking, and injecting the drug to get the quickest high at the cheapest cost.

I asked if she had thoughts of suicide. She told me no, that she was too close to her mom and her younger sister. "I'm glad you came in," I told her, seeking a positive note.

She kept crying, her despair soon enveloping her entire body with racking coughs. Rebecca, who had initially called me to see Natalie, heard the noise and came in the room.

"Everything okay?" she asked.

Natalie grasped her stomach again. "I think I'm going to be sick."

Rebecca looked at me. "I think we should get her something to help her right now."

At the time, management of opioid withdrawal, from what I'd seen around the hospital, involved what we called *symptomatic treatment*. That meant medicines to limit diarrhea, ease nausea, and soothe muscle cramps. We also gave a blood pressure drug called clonidine that helped calm the underlying cause of withdrawal—a hyperactive nervous system—and thus reduced symptoms globally. A newer drug, buprenorphine, which later became a central treatment for people like Natalie, required a special certification to prescribe, so very few doctors in the general hospital setting could issue it. Methadone, an older drug, was even more restricted.

"We'll be right back," Rebecca said to Natalie.

We stepped out of the room and walked to a computer workstation area where I began entering orders. Craig, the charge nurse, joined us.

"Did she tell you about what happened during her deployment?" Rebecca asked me.

I shook my head. I didn't yet know she'd been deployed. In psychiatry, as compared to general medicine and surgery, we were expected to get a lot more of the "social history"—details about work, education, relationships, and the like. During daytime hours, I enjoyed learning these aspects about my patients' lives—but at 4:30 A.M., I wanted only the bare facts.

"Where was she deployed?" I asked.

At the VA hospital, military history took on particular importance, given the high prevalence of Vietnam veterans and the influx of young veterans from Iraq and Afghanistan that we were beginning to see. Rebecca told me that Natalie had been deployed to the Middle East on a combat assignment, but it wasn't nightmares of rocket attacks and road-side bombs that tortured her.

"She was assaulted," Rebecca said. "Drugged and raped."

It all made sense—her reluctance to talk with me alone, and her request to keep the door open while we did. What happened to Natalie was widespread enough that national VA headquarters had already given it a label—military sexual trauma, or MST for short. Craig seethed as Rebecca provided some of the sordid details of her attack.

"I wish that guy was right here so I could beat the shit out of him," he said.

I felt a similar impulse. But I needed to focus on the here and now. I scanned through her electronic chart and saw that her lab results had returned. Normal kidney and liver function. Normal electrolyte values. Normal blood cell counts. Her urine drug screen indicated recent opioid use; it showed no signals for any of the other drugs we tested.

"So what are you thinking as far as your plan?" Rebecca asked me.

In the emergency room, whether the primary issue is medical, surgical, or psychiatric, the thinking is essentially the same: the patient either goes "out" (discharged or transferred) or "up" (admitted). Sometimes there is a gray area of "observation" that buys more time to make that call. But with Natalie, the data was all essentially in place. Her lab tests were fine. Her vital signs were only slightly abnormal. She reported no suicidal ideation whatsoever, and we had nothing to refute that: She'd come to our hospital on her own without coercion. She didn't show any sign of being manic or psychotic. Hers seemed to be a straightforward case of what we referred to then as *opioid dependence*, and the protocol I'd been told was that those cases were managed on an outpatient basis. That meant she needed to be sent "out," with a plan for clinic-based aftercare.

I shared that news with the nurses, and that's when Craig erupted, questioning my judgment. After all, we admitted alcohol and cocaine "users" all the time. They were invariably men, it seemed, and most much older. Here we had a young woman, one who'd been viciously assaulted in the military and was now in the early stages of a drug problem initially triggered by a doctor's prescription. She presented to us in clear distress and sought our help, and the best we could offer was to send her out in the darkness of a Saturday morning with a plan that someone would call her in two days, at the earliest, to schedule an appointment? Put that way, it sounded flimsy, but I was pretty certain that this was going to be our treatment outcome. I left the nursing station and went to a workroom where I paged my supervisor, Dr. Reid.

"Hello, Damon," he said, his voice groggy.

Dr. Reid was the senior psychiatrist on duty at the hospital for the entire weekend, Friday evening through Monday morning. He had to see all new hospital admissions and discuss with us residents any patients discharged from the emergency room. He'd been a resident in our program several years earlier, and was generally sympathetic to the challenges we faced. I explained Natalie's case to him.

"No suicidal behaviors at all?" he asked. "Past or present?"

In emergency psychiatry, assessing suicide risk often took primacy over every other consideration. We got information from medical records, from the patient, from family and friends, and, in some instances, from physical signs of self-inflicted injury. Natalie had no data in her medical chart, denied suicidal thoughts, and given that she'd sought help as an adult woman who lived alone, it didn't seem necessary to involve family or friends. At least not at a quarter to five on a Saturday morning.

To my mind, injecting heroin constituted its own form of self-injury, given that it increased risks for various life-threatening infections, but it wasn't considered such in the framework I'd been taught. Her self-reported intention wasn't to cause death or disability; rather, she sought to block out emotional distress from her past and, as time wore on, to blunt the effects of being in opioid withdrawal. I explained all this to Dr. Reid.

"Sounds like we're dealing with PTSD and opioid dependence," he concluded.

I described my conversation with the nurses and explained to him my reservations about sending her home with a plan for someone to call her to set up a clinic appointment. I asked if we could make an exception and admit her to our psychiatric unit.

"Her situation is very sad," Dr. Reid said, "but you have to take into account that admitting her to our unit upstairs—the way it's set up—might actually worsen her PTSD."

I hadn't considered that point, although it was obvious now that he'd mentioned it. More than 90 percent of the patients on the psychiatry unit then—on many days, all the patients—were male, with shared rooms and a common bathroom for the entire floor. The unit had a few single rooms to house frail elderly people, particularly disruptive patients, or women. But even with her own room and private bathroom, Natalie might have wound up the only woman on a floor with twenty-five men in various states of psychological distress, some with a history of questionable behavior toward women.

"Maybe she could be admitted to general medicine?" I wondered aloud, then quickly realized this wasn't a viable option based on my recent experience as an intern on that unit; the general medicine services then regarded opioid misuse primarily as a psychiatric problem.

"Not with her lab numbers and vital signs," Dr. Reid answered.

Dr. Reid then mentioned a community crisis center where we sometimes sent patients who showed up at our university hospitals with drug and alcohol problems.

I'd already considered that option, but they served only residents of our local county. Natalie lived just across the county line, in a smaller one with fewer resources. I informed Dr. Reid.

"Well, it looks like the best we can offer her is a referral to our outpatient substance abuse treatment program," he said. "There's really no better option."

It was predawn on Saturday morning, and no one would have access to outpatient schedules until Monday, more than forty-eight hours later. At that point, a medical clerk, in between checking in arriving patients, would call Natalie to set up an appointment that might take place later that week. Or the next. And this assumed that our request was received and processed under a best-case response, and not buried underneath a backlog of paperwork from the previous week.

Our plan was set. Now it was time to break the news to everyone. I started with the nurses.

"They need something intermediate, between outpatient and what's upstairs," Rebecca said to me. "There's going to be more and more people like her over time."

"I can't believe how bad our services are," Craig said, shaking his head. "This girl goes to Iraq and has bad things happen to her, and this is the best we can do for her?"

Actually, when it came to treating people with drug-related problems, the VA was certainly no worse than any other setting where I'd worked. If anything, they had more resources available, in both hospital and clinic settings. The fact that those services were nonetheless inadequate at the time was a broader reflection of how substance use was marginalized by general physicians, medical specialists, and psychiatrists alike.

Rebecca accompanied me as I went to update Natalie. Outside her door, an old man on a stretcher was whisked past us, wheeled by a nurse to the radiology area, probably for a CT scan. He wore a breathing mask that pumped oxygen through his nostrils. It reminded me that the ER wasn't the best place to treat emotional distress.

Natalie was lying down on her back. She tensely sat up as we entered. Slowly, I laid out the thinking that had gone into her case. Then I braced myself for a tongue-lashing about how VA hospitals didn't care about vets, as some had told me, or how doctors or nurses were only in it for the money, as others had said. Whatever Craig had offered in the way of disapproval, I expected Natalie's reaction to be worse. Instead, she glanced down briefly, wiped away a few tears, and then looked up at us.

"Thanks for doing everything you could," she said. "And for talking to me."

I was tongue-tied. My time on hospital wards, in emergency rooms, and in outpatient clinics had largely reinforced negative messages about substance-using patients: Irresponsible. Needy. Ungrateful. We invariably saw them in their worst moments, rather than in settings demonstrating their various strengths and potential for change. Some doctors we worked alongside were full of condescending judgment, despite lectures we'd all received on the biological mechanisms of addiction, and the incontrovertible reality of doctors' elevated risks for alcohol and drug problems. Natalie's story, however, forced me to reconsider the complexity of how addiction could take root and disrupt someone's life. And to recognize our clear shortcomings in treating it.

I confirmed Natalie's phone number and mailing address in our system and told her that someone from our outpatient substance abuse treatment program would contact her early the following week to schedule an appointment.

"How long will it take for me to be seen there?" she asked.

"Probably within a week or two," I said, struck by the limitations of a plan to send her back out to the same environment where she'd struggled for months after only a half-hour conversation.

In the interim, we gave her a few days' worth of "symptom-based" pills to ease her withdrawal symptoms and hoped that, with those anti-nausea, anti-diarrhea, and anti-inflammatory pills, she could avoid the desire to obtain Vicodin, Percocet, OxyContin, or heroin. Although our plan met the "standard of care" then, it nonetheless felt as if we had not fulfilled our duties. Maybe I should have gotten her family involved before discharging her? Or fudged her address so that the local crisis center would take her? And even though I could not have prescribed either drug to her that night, why hadn't we even talked about methadone or buprenorphine as treatment options?

IN 2002, A FEW YEARS BEFORE I MET NATALIE, THE FDA APPROVED a drug called buprenorphine as a treatment for opioid use disorder. When I transferred into the psychiatry program, one of the first lectures I recall was hearing a psychiatrist at our hospital tell a group of us residents how this medication would revolutionize opioid treatment. He said that it was one of the most important advances ever in addiction medicine. Media coverage was equally enthusiastic.

Before then, methadone programs had been the primary medication therapy for opioid (mainly heroin) dependence since the 1970s. But methadone had several limitations. Patients were required by federal and state laws to attend a clinic, often every day, where they might have to wait in lines for supervised administration of their medicine. Many clinics were located in isolated, lower-income areas that operated completely outside the traditional medical system. As a result, most doctors, psychiatrists included, never saw the inside of an Opioid Treatment Program, as they are officially named. We didn't really know what went on there; what we did know was that when patients on methadone arrived at our clinics and hospitals, we wanted to address their medical issue as quickly as possible and send them back where they would be out of sight again.

Buprenorphine held the promise to reform this widespread marginalization of opioid treatment, as it could be prescribed in an outpatient clinic in same location where a psychiatrist treats depression and panic disorder, or a primary care provider manages diabetes, hypertension, and high cholesterol. From there, the patient could go to a conventional pharmacy and receive up to a one-month supply rather than make a daily trek to a special clinic. Buprenorphine was going to bring opioid treatment out of the darkness and into the mainstream.

But that didn't really happen. Although it was easier to prescribe than methadone, doctors still had to submit to numerous restrictions when prescribing (for example, completion of a special eight-hour course, and a cap on the number of patients one could treat). These rules made buprenorphine seem particularly dangerous, an ironic outcome given that opioid pain medication, for which people sought care from the clutches of addiction, could be ordered with limited scrutiny by a medical intern. These prescribing barriers, along with the enduring stigma of addiction as a moral failing rather than a medical illness, resulted in about 8 percent of eligible physicians obtaining the waiver to dispense buprenorphine as of 2019. And even within this eligible group, few actually prescribed this drug to patients.

"Treating people with addiction can be complicated," Dr. Joseph Lee, president and CEO of the Hazelden Betty Ford Foundation, told me. "So expecting doctors to fit that into a fifteen-minute visit while managing a host of other health problems isn't really realistic. We need to think about how we structure our health system if we really want to address it."

The COVID-19 pandemic, with the social and occupational dislocations it wrought, made the problem with opioids and other drugs even worse. With fentanyl flooding the market of nonprescription opioid use, US overdose deaths related to opioids skyrocketed in 2020, increasing from nearly fifty thousand the prior year to seventy thousand. In 2021, opioid-related deaths topped eighty thousand. Preliminary data suggests these rates may have increased even further in 2022.

In December 2022, as opioid deaths continued to surge amid a waning pandemic, the federal government took its most assertive steps yet: with bipartisan passage of the Consolidated Appropriations Act, 2023, they eliminated the requirement for a special eight-hour training as well as the rigid cap on how many patients a doctor could treat with buprenorphine at any one time. Essentially, any doctor can now prescribe this medicine to treat opioid addiction. But with the stigma that attends treating drug-related matters, the impact of these reforms, while undoubtedly a positive development, remains an open question.

"This is an important and necessary step," Dr. Lee said of the recent policy changes. "But we also have to find a way to encourage more good people to enter this field, so we can do a better job of translating what we know works in theory into clinical practice."

Dr. Lee spoke of how the month he spent working at a residential treatment facility during his psychiatry residency changed his outlook on addiction treatment. There, he had the time to interact with patients as "whole people in recovery" rather than seeing them in the crisis mode that dominated medical education.

"I think if more doctors got that sort of exposure to addiction medicine earlier in their training, to the kind of hope and transformation that happens every day," he told me, "medicine would be doing a better job addressing addiction."

His comments made me reflect on my education and mindset toward addiction when I met Natalie that night in the ER. I had a vague sense then that buprenorphine, along with psychological care, could be an appropriate treatment for her, but I lacked the knowledge to discuss this with her thoughtfully. As psychiatry residents, we had a one-month

addiction psychiatry requirement scheduled at a later stage in our training. The thirty-minute lecture from the buprenorphine enthusiast months
earlier got lost in the thicket of busy shifts trying to learn the diagnostic jargon and medications we used on a regular basis. The primary ER
doctor that night when Natalie came in wasn't a full-time emergency
physician but rather a medical subspecialist moonlighting in the ER to
pay off his medical school loans, so he knew even less than I did about
treating opioid withdrawal. If you had chest pain or lung problems,
he knew exactly what to do, just as I knew by memory the protocol for
treating alcohol withdrawal or a manic episode; yet we would have both
struggled with any serious test that measured our up-to-date knowledge
on opioid withdrawal management.

Natalie represented my introduction, in a direct and tangible way, to
the world of opioid addiction. I'd been a doctor for more than a year, with
two additional clinical years in medical school. Yet at that point, I'd only
dealt with patients whose opioid misuse was a secondary issue to some
more urgent medical concern. Or at least that was the way I had inter-
preted those situations. But in just a matter of weeks, my experiences
encountering people with opioid problems would rapidly accelerate. The
results were harrowing.

A FEW HOURS AFTER NATALIE LEFT, MY TWENTY-FOUR-HOUR SHIFT
was done, and with it, a stretch of months at the VA hospital. I spent the
next four weeks at Duke on the hospital-based psychiatry consult service,
where we fielded requests from other doctors. General medicine teams
asked us to determine if someone had the requisite mental capacity to
refuse various treatments. Surgeons wanted our help managing people
acutely confused in the days following an operation. Neurologists sought
our input for patients who arrived with seizure-like episodes or widespread weakness that couldn't be explained by physical exam, EEG, or
MRI. The OB-GYN team called us to see women whose current behavior raised alarms for carrying the pregnancy to term or raising the
child afterward.

I enjoyed the work, as it gave me the opportunity to blend my psychiatry training with the years of medical internship and medical school that preceded it. But the hours were taxing; we often stayed until well after 6:00 P.M. during the week and also worked some emergency department shifts on weekends. In the throes of this hectic pace, and the wide swath of patients I encountered, I soon forgot about Natalie. About midway through this rotation, however, I received a page that brought her back to my conscious thoughts.

I had just finished seeing an older man with pancreatitis who was having bad alcohol withdrawal when my pager buzzed. I'd been sent a text message: *"We have a consult for you in the MICU."*

My chest tightened briefly. It was barely 9:00 A.M., and I already had three new consults. My coresident was away all morning at his clinic. The day before had been unusually calm and quiet, with just two straightforward consults between us; it seemed we were being punished as a result. This was my first time getting a consult from the medical ICU, and the unknown was invariably unsettling to me.

"Psych consult pager, this is Dr. Tweedy," I said after dialing the return number.

"Hey, Damon, this is Elliot."

Elliot was a second-year general medicine resident. We'd started internal medicine residency together before I switched over to psychiatry at the end of that first year.

"How is psych going?" he asked.

I hesitated. While I believed that I'd made a good decision for my own life and career in changing programs, a part of me still felt awkward around former colleagues and supervisors. I carried a nagging sense that, in various ways practical and symbolic, I had let them down. The mindset of being "a tough soldier" was hard to relinquish.

"Good," I said, blandly. "How's second year for you?"

"It's better than last year," he answered. "Although MICU is a beast."

For a brief moment, I imagined days and nights filled with code blue resuscitations and central venous line insertions. Those aspects of doctoring were mostly gone forever in my life, and that suited me fine.

"What do you have for me?" I asked.

"We've got a young woman who's been here three days. Bad OD. Heroin and alprazolam."

Alprazolam, better known as Xanax, belonged to a class of sedatives, benzodiazepines, which I was quickly learning were lifesaving for some people but life-threatening for many others—especially when combined with alcohol or opioids.

"We just extubated her yesterday afternoon," Elliot continued. "At the beginning, we didn't think she would make it. And that even if she did, she might have brain damage."

But miraculously, he told me, she seemed to have retained normal brain function, at least the parts that controlled consciousness, speech, and physical movements. Psychologically, however, she seemed despondent. Elliot and the rest of the medical team wanted our input to sort out whether her overdose was accidental or a genuine suicide attempt. The former meant she could probably go home after another day of medical observation; the latter would likely necessitate transfer to an inpatient psychiatric unit.

Five minutes later, I stood outside the room of my new patient, Brandy. I'd walked past several ICU rooms on the way there, each with a large bed in the center housing a very sick person: tubes projecting from varied body parts, monitors generating continuous data. But Brandy's bed was empty. A thirtyish nurse sat in a high chair outside her room, a portable computer workstation directly in front of her. I introduced myself.

"She's in the bathroom," she said. "She really needs you."

I nodded. Nurses and doctors on medical and surgical services often told me this when they sent us consults. But I was still less than a year removed from working in the ICU and medical wards myself. I certainly did not feel like a mental health expert.

"Her situation is really sad," she continued. "Especially since she's got a young daughter."

My instinct was to judge Brandy harshly. How could a mom of a small kid use drugs? But I quickly swatted away those thoughts. After all, at the time, I had no children and could never become pregnant. My life was mostly good. Could I really stand in judgment of hers?

"Hopefully, we can help get her on a good track," I said.

I used the time waiting for her to skim through her medical chart in the break room, and soon found myself engrossed by the details in her medical admission note. Brandy's drug problems had started in the aftermath of a serious car accident where she'd sustained a wrist fracture and torn shoulder ligament. A doctor prescribed an opioid drug while her injuries healed. He later gave her alprazolam to help with panic attacks and insomnia that stemmed from the accident. Before long, she was taking excess amounts of both and, after some months, escalated from prescription pain pills to heroin.

My eyes remained glued to the page, but my mind had shifted its focus elsewhere. Suddenly, I found myself replaying the overnight VA encounter with Natalie from weeks earlier. Brandy's story, both in how her opioid use started and how it escalated, sounded similar to Natalie's. I then thought back to my most recent experience taking opioids after knee surgery: after a few days, I eagerly stopped the nausea-inducing pills once the pain became tolerable. Again, I pondered what accounted for the difference between my reaction to these drugs and the reaction of the patients whose lives they consumed.

I didn't hear the nurse enter the room or see her approach me.

"She's ready," she told me.

I flinched, dropping the pen I'd been holding. For a brief moment, I'd lost track of my surroundings.

"Everything okay?" the nurse asked.

I assured her that I was simply tired, but she didn't seem totally convinced. Her confidence in me helping Brandy seemed to wane a bit.

I hurried over to Brandy's bedside. Her face looked ghost pale, surrounded by platinum-blond hair. I introduced myself and tried to make some awkward small talk before homing in on the central question that needed to be addressed.

"I had a chance to read your chart," I began, "and I know you've been through a lot. Do you remember what your thoughts were before you over-dosed? Were you attempting to kill yourself? Or was it something else?"

Her eyes met mine briefly, then she looked away, her voice soft, mono-tone, and distant: "I don't know, honestly."

"How do you feel now that you're . . . that you are still alive?" I asked.

I'd seen some patients who survived suicide attempts convincingly state that this experience gave them a new, more positive outlook on life. But everyone didn't enjoy such transformation: a previous suicide attempt is a big risk factor for a later completed suicide.

"I'm not sure," she said. "I shouldn't have done it. Now I'm going to lose my girl."

I didn't know if that was true, nor was it my job to get involved with that decision. Based on her responses, coupled with the seriousness of her overdose, Brandy appeared in need of transfer to a psychiatric unit. She had Medicaid, which limited her available options, but we'd find her a bed. I was determined. She seemed more depressed than Natalie. Was that because she was further along in her drug addiction? I wondered if a doctor had effectively "turned her away from treatment" at an earlier stage of care like I felt I'd done with Natalie, and that her overdose was the near-tragic consequence. In my mind, I had to make this situation right by Brandy to atone for Natalie, even though I didn't know what that meant exactly.

I continued to think about both women throughout the day despite the steady patient flow and afternoon rounds with our supervisor that spilled into the early evening. The next morning, our psychiatry pro-gram held its weekly academic half day, where each class of residents (years one through four) had a variety of educational seminars designed for their level of training. It also provided a much-needed chance to so-cialize in short bursts, since we were spread across several hospitals and clinics and would otherwise not see each other.

During a brief break between lectures, Nelson, one of my coresidents, approached me. Instead of the usual "How is it going at X location or with X attending?" or "When is your next vacation?" greeting, he brought up a specific patient.

"Do you remember Mr. Frost?" he asked. "The guy with anxiety and drug abuse we had on our services at the VA? The one who seemed like he had borderline PD?"

For reasons that were at least somewhat sexist, women were far more likely than men to get the diagnosis of borderline personality disorder, a label whose stigma within psychiatry and general medicine was on par with those who misused drugs. A man with both diagnoses tended to stand out for the medical staff, mostly for the worse.

"Sure," I responded. "What about him?"

I'm not sure what exactly I expected Nelson to say. Maybe that Mr. Frost had gotten readmitted again. Or lodged a formal complaint to some administrative person asserting that we were incompetent doctors. Despite the many red flags an outside observer might have noted in his medical record, I was wholly unprepared for what Nelson told me.

"He OD'd two days ago."

"What?" I asked, stunned.

He'd been admitted to our psychiatric unit two months earlier after an argument with his on-again, off-again girlfriend where he'd threatened to cut his wrists, get behind the wheel, and submerge his car in a nearby lake. But they reconciled a few days into his hospital stay, and his suicidal impulses subsided.

"He took a cocktail of opioids. Oxycodone, hydrocodone, and something else."

"Is he . . ."

"He's dead," Nelson said, his eyes searching my face, a look of pain on his own. "His girlfriend found him in their bedroom."

We'd both had patients die while we worked on general medicine teams. But this felt different. Mr. Frost was in his early thirties, barely older than we were, and unlike someone that age who had a tragic case of terminal cancer, his death felt somehow preventable.

"Damn," I said, disbelieving.

By his third day in the hospital on my inpatient team, Mr. Frost started asking for opioids for low back pain; we refused, and the following morning he requested discharge. He'd been readmitted to Nelson's team the following week with similar demands. What had we missed? Could he have been in opioid withdrawal that we failed to recognize?

"How'd you find out?" I asked.

"She called the ER to report what happened, and apparently, they got Dr. Morrison on the phone. She proceeded to curse him out pretty bad."

A sense of dread spread through me. Dr. Morrison was a senior psychiatrist. He was going to comb through the medical chart and see our notes. Nelson read my mind:

"I looked through his records last night. He came back to the ER after he left my service. So it's not like either of us were the last people to see him."

Still, even if no reprimands were coming our way, we both felt helpless. We were late to the start of the next seminar, and I struggled to focus the rest of the morning. During the lunch hour, I passed on catching up with colleagues and rushed across the street to the VA hospital to log on to their medical record system. Between hearing of Mr. Frost's fatal overdose and witnessing the aftermath of Brandy's near-death episode, I had to find out what happened with Natalie. I needed to follow up on my ER encounter with her, to see if my referral had gone through as hoped.

I jogged to an upstairs overnight call room, knowing it would be vacant this time of day. In my haste, I failed to log in on my first two attempts. One more failure and I would be locked out for at least an hour.

"Damn it," I said aloud.

It had been a few weeks since I'd logged in, long enough for me to forget my password. On the third try, I closed my eyes and gently touched the keys in a sequence familiar to me, muscle memory at work. It felt right, so I pressed the "Enter" key and held my breath. A yellow square appeared in the center of the screen, indicating that I had successfully accessed the record system. I had no problem recalling Natalie's full name; within seconds, her chart came into focus.

My pulse raced as I stared at the files. My physician note from her ER visit, the one from nearly three weeks before, was the last entry in her chart.

I clicked on the tab labeled "consults." My order had been processed.

An administrative clerk from the substance abuse treatment program had called Natalie. Twice. The first time, she noted that she'd left a voicemail; the second time she'd received an automated reply that the mailbox was full and could not receive additional messages. She then sent a letter requesting Natalie to call the clinic; so far, it had gone unanswered.

I felt beads of sweat along my forehead. I picked up the nearby phone and started to dial Natalie's number. But I stopped myself before finishing. What would happen if she actually picked up? Would she remember me? And if she did, would her initial gratitude have turned sour? What if her mom picked up, told me she was still using, and yelled at me for not doing more for her daughter when she'd driven thirty miles in the middle of the night for our help? Maybe these were all excuses for my own cowardice. In the end, I put down the phone, logged out of the medical record system, and clumsily walked across the street to the other hospital to resume the rest of my day.

WHAT WOULD BE DIFFERENT IF NATALIE HAD SHOWN UP TODAY? TO help me answer that question, I reached out to a few professional colleagues who've made treating addiction a core mission of their work lives. Drs. Dana Clifton and Noel Ivey lead a program at Duke called COMET, where the goal is to initiate medications in hospital for patients with opioid use disorder and improve their transition into the community after discharge.

"Her scenario was very common back then," Dr. Clifton said, referring to Natalie. "We would treat the medical complications of opioid use disorder and injection drug use—systemic infections, such as bacteremia or endocarditis, for example—but not usually address the underlying condition, which was their drug use."

Dr. Clifton's frustration with the status quo led her and Dr. Ivey to implement a program where general internal medicine physicians are trained to provide patients opioid withdrawal treatment in the hospital, while being paired with clinical social workers who can help the patients get set for care outside the hospital.

"Someone like your patient," Dr. Ivey said, "they would get buprenor-phine in the ER. That would be the starting point."

In many ERs nowadays, she'd also get a take-home Narcan (nalox-one) kit to reverse a potential overdose. And test strips to help her avoid fentanyl, which is much more lethal than heroin. Both locally, where I saw Natalie, and nationally, emergency rooms are also nowadays better equipped to set patients up with programs to continue buprenorphine (or start methadone), and get them into counseling for ongoing treatment. If these resources had been in place then, sending Natalie home would not have felt so dispiriting.

None of these efforts would have promised a cure for Natalie, of course. Or even a good outcome. The same uncertainty was true for the patients who came to us with heart attacks, colon cancer, or an assort-ment of other medical conditions. But having the ability to provide the best available care to someone in need, to ease their distress without causing further harm, this was what good doctoring was all about. That was what Natalie deserved.

MY SCHEDULE REMAINED BUSY DURING THE ENSUING MONTHS, AND over time, as I endured a barbaric stretch at the state hospital, certain details about Natalie started to fade from my memory. I forgot her last name and her medical record number, so I couldn't access her chart the next time I returned to the VA hospital. Nor did I have legitimate rea-son to do so then; by that point, Natalie was no longer my patient, and our encounter had officially been closed.

But the essence of our interaction remained vivid. Each time I'd see or hear about a patient who misused opioids—and they soon came in large numbers—I thought of Natalie and wondered how she was doing. Had she eventually found her way into our outpatient system and got-ten the treatment she needed, or had she sought care elsewhere? Did she stop on her own? Or was she still using? If so, had she become entangled with the legal system along the way? Or did she die from an overdose, like Mr. Frost, and over 550,000 other people between 1999 and 2020? I would never know these answers. Perhaps that was best.

What remained clear was that general medicine and psychiatry had done much to worsen the epidemic of opioids, benzodiazepines, and other drugs with considerable risk for addiction, but too often then treated the patients involved with disdain. Doctors, clinics, and hospitals shared the blame, but so did pharmaceutical companies, politicians, and health insurance companies. The first several months of my psychiatric training reinforced that while stigma was nearly universal for those with mental illness, people with drug-related problems occupied a separate location beneath all others—a space where we most often failed patients.

6

FROM HEAD TO TOE

LENNIE SOBBED AS THE SURGEONS BROKE THE NEWS. HIS MIND flashed back to when he was a football and track star in high school three decades earlier. Now he didn't know when he would be able to walk again, much less run. Even if he did eventually reach those goals, it would never be the same. Not even close. His doctors had just told him that his left foot and lower left leg needed to be amputated.

Our paths crossed forty-eight hours later, on a cool and rainy Wednesday morning. Lennie had undergone his operation the previous day, and while it had saved the rest of his leg, and quite possibly his life, he wasn't in the mood for gratitude. But he wasn't depressed either, at least not in the tearful or despondent way people often are in his situation. Instead, he was angry. Furious. He wanted vengeance.

"He told the nurse he wants to hurt the people who put him in this position," said Sanjeev, the surgical resident who'd called me.

After three months working at the state psychiatric facility twenty minutes away, I was back at our main university medical campus for another stint on the hospital consult service. There, we fielded psychiatric calls from different clinical departments throughout the medical center. This one came just as I'd finished with another patient.

"Who is he blaming?" I asked Sanjeev, trying to gauge whether Lennie's wrath presented an urgent threat or something less acute.

Most people faced with terrible health misfortunes point the finger at someone for their circumstances. Some blame themselves for not taking care of their bodies sooner. Others blame outside forces—the driver who crashed into them, the boss who overworked them, the cigarette or drug company that withheld information on their product's dangers. Still others look further outward, far beyond their immediate lives, to God for forsaking them, the devil for tempting them, or a politician whom they dislike for simply being in office.

"At first," Sanjeev began, "the nurse thought he was mad at us, you know, for doing the amputation, even though he accepted that it was needed."

Medicine was rife with violent acts done in the name of helping a patient. Perhaps none was as visceral as literally severing a limb.

"But it's not us," Sanjeev continued. "He's mad at the doctors who treated him at the other hospitals before he was transferred here."

Sanjeev explained that Lennie had initially gone to an emergency room with two concerns: severe depression and foot pain. But once he mentioned feeling hopeless, he believed the doctors focused only on that problem. They sent him to a psychiatry hospital, and he spent more than a day there before a doctor came to look at his foot.

"So he thinks someone should have caught the problem sooner," I summarized.

"Exactly. He said they didn't listen to him. And he says that's why his foot and lower leg got so bad we had to cut them off."

"Well, I see why he's so upset," I said.

As compelling as the story was, it wasn't clear to me what the surgeons wanted from our psychiatry team. The emergency room where he'd first been seen was twenty minutes away, and the psychiatric hospital even farther. Just twenty-four hours from his amputation, he wasn't going anywhere for a while. Were they concerned he might turn his rage inward and hurt himself in his hospital bed?

"He denied that," Sanjeev answered. "Categorically."

"Are you afraid he's going to sabotage his own recovery in some other way?"

"No," Sanjeev replied. "He seems very motivated. Like he's fueled in an angry way."

"Is he yelling or cursing at any of your staff?"

"No, nothing like that. He's been respectful to everyone here. He's laser-focused on getting better. But he's really mad at those other doctors. That's what makes us nervous."

"Since he's not going to leave the hospital or get around for a while," I said, "is there any reason he needs to be seen today? Or could this wait until he's closer to discharge?"

I wasn't trying to avoid seeing him; rather, I wanted to use my time efficiently. Some consults had to be seen on the spot—a medically unstable patient urgently trying to leave the hospital, for example—whereas others could be triaged for later. We had other patients to visit, so I couldn't see why Lennie should jump the line. But Sanjeev's next words made me reconsider.

"My attending wanted us to call the police when he heard about the threats, but I persuaded him to let me call you all first."

Sanjeev told me that Lennie had a criminal record, according to the notes from the other hospital. But details were fuzzy. Regardless, calling the police seemed extreme given his physical state. He might end up hating our doctors as much as he did the others.

Sanjeev kept on: "I've seen you guys help people. Maybe there is something you can recommend that would calm him down a bit more. Or maybe you could just talk to him to make sure we're not missing something. This isn't our expertise."

I looked at the printed list of patients that our team was following. Our morning was full. Adding Lennie to the mix meant I might need to work through lunch, grabbing one of those hospital-issued liquid supplements on the go. Yuck. But my mind played the image of a man being interrogated by police and cuffed to his handrail less than a day after losing his foot and part of his leg. My dietary preferences would have to be an afterthought.

"There's one person I have to see right now," I said. "It shouldn't take too long. I'll be there in twenty minutes. Thirty minutes, tops."

———

BY THIS POINT IN TRAINING, EARLY IN MY SECOND YEAR AS A psychiatry resident and third overall as a doctor, I knew that having a psychiatric illness led to worse health outcomes for people. Suicide was the obvious example, but I also saw how mental illness led to various unintended problems, some fatal, others chronically disabling. A widely discussed 2006 report from the federal government's Center for Mental Health Services expanded the conversation further, revealing that people with psychiatric disorders in the public health system died fifteen to thirty years earlier than those in the rest of the population. More striking, they observed that the leading causes of death were not suicide or accidental overdose, but heart disease, cancer, stroke, and lung diseases. As the authors concluded, "People with mental illness have medical problems that lead to death, especially if they have inadequate medical treatment." Put more simply, having a serious mental malady was bad for your physical health.

While some doctors stress the role that society plays in these medical disparities—rising income inequality and state budget cuts for mental health care, for example—most conversations I heard then around poorer health outcomes came back to individual behavior. People with psychiatric disorders as a whole are less likely to follow standard medical recommendations, missing clinic appointments and leaving prescriptions unfilled. They are likelier to misuse substances, have less nutritious diets, and lead more sedentary lives. Their sleep patterns are often highly irregular. In most cases, a patient with a psychiatric illness will score worse on these "health behaviors" than an otherwise similar person.

What wasn't discussed nearly as much in my training was the role that we as doctors and other medical providers played in these adverse outcomes. Occasionally, we acknowledged that a subset of the medications we prescribed—especially those for bipolar disorder and schizophrenia—could cause significant weight gain and other adverse health effects, but often those were considered unfortunate side effects that nevertheless served the greater good for the patient, who otherwise would suffer far greater from their mental distress. In that regard, we compared ourselves to oncologists treating cancer. Our treatments could be toxic, but without them, the patient would be worse off. As a busy novice in the field, I felt unqualified to question that perspective.

But what struck me, even at this early stage, was how differently many doctors perceived physical health complaints when a patient had a significant psychiatric illness. Too often, they saw the label on a chart—or perceived that the patient in front of them had psychological troubles—and it became the smoking gun that solved the case. Leads pointing to other potential suspects were effectively cast aside.

One evening during my internship year, our medical team got a call from the emergency department about an admission: a fiftysomething-year-old woman with sudden-onset chest pain. Her EKG was inconclusive for a heart attack or other acute heart problems, so the emergency medicine resident wanted to send her upstairs for further monitoring and serial blood testing. At first blush, this sounded like a bread-and-butter case. I sat next to Kyle, the resident on our service, in our workroom as he spoke with this doctor. Kyle put the call on speaker so he wouldn't have to waste time relaying the information to me later.

"What's her medical record number?" Kyle asked.

He pulled up the woman's electronic medical chart as the ER resident spoke. Chest pain cases were among the most straightforward problems we saw. If her blood tests indicated a heart attack, we would consult the cardiology team to help manage her care. If not, we could order a few additional tests and get her set up for an outpatient appointment with her primary care doctor. Either way, she wouldn't stay on our service for long. Kyle knew this even better than I did, so I was surprised when he began interrogating this doctor, who was at the same level of training as he was.

"I see that she has a history of depression and anxiety," Kyle said. "What makes you think this isn't just a panic attack?"

Along with chest pain, panic attacks can have other symptoms, such as difficulty breathing, nausea, and sweating, that overlap with heart attacks. Millions of people come to hospitals each year with chest pain, a sizable number due to panic attacks.

"She says the pain started while she was exercising," the ER resident replied, "which makes me think it could be cardiac and not simply psychological. And she said she was doing okay stress-wise."

Kyle and the ER resident went back and forth on the presence or absence of various cardiac risk factors for this woman before the ER resident lost his patience.

"Look," he said, sounding exasperated, "if you all want to discharge her as soon as she gets upstairs, that's your prerogative. But we're not going to sign off on sending her home based on the information we have here. I can get my supervisor on the phone if you want to hear it from her."

Kyle seethed as he disconnected the call. "This person shouldn't be sent to us now," he said, rubbing his eyes so hard I worried he might bruise them. "She's on Prozac, Wellbutrin, and Xanax. Three psych drugs. She probably just needs a psychiatrist to adjust her meds or to go talk with a psychologist."

We were in the midst of a bad week, our team list filled with complicated patients. Still, Kyle had mostly remained poised and thoughtful in addressing their medical issues and pleasant when talking with them at their bedside. Yet somehow this woman's mental health history triggered a reflex to discount her medical symptoms. Perhaps he assumed that her psychiatric diagnoses meant that she was exaggerating her physical concern. One of my previous female supervisors had told me that women in general were more likely to have their worries dismissed in this way, but Kyle had generally seemed open-minded with our patients, male and female alike. Maybe he would have felt differently had he had a chance to see and talk with her along with the ER resident. In a different hospital without close faculty supervision, though, and with a less confident doctor on the other end, Kyle might have pressured emergency medical staff to send this woman home without laying eyes on her.

Thankfully, that didn't happen. It turned out this woman hadn't had a heart attack. But an upper endoscopy procedure showed some damage to her esophagus. While it wasn't life-threatening like a heart attack and ultimately could be treated on an outpatient basis, this condition did explain her chest pain symptoms. The ER doctor had been correct; it wasn't just "all in her head," and it had been worthwhile to make sure that her heart was functioning well. Throughout her hospital stay, Kyle went out of his way to be nice to her. He probably felt bad about his initial impression of her, formed by her medical chart.

When I switched to psychiatry, I found that medical problems were sometimes neglected there too. On one occasion, our team accepted a sixty-year-old man with schizophrenia from a local mental health facility for a recurrence of delusional speech and behaviors. As he passed through the ER on his way upstairs to our psychiatric unit, the ER physician suggested to my supervisor that day, a psychiatrist a few years out of training, that we check a urine sample to make sure he didn't have an infection in his urinary tract, as the patient had urinated on himself prior to arrival. Urine infections were a known cause of confusion in older patients, but the outside facility hadn't obtained a sample for testing.

It was near the end of the regular workday, and I got the sense that the psychiatrist wanted to get everything tidied up with the admission orders as quickly as possible.

"We can get our nurses upstairs to get a sample tomorrow," he said.

The ER doctor frowned. "It's easier for us to get it down here with our nurses," she said, matter-of-factly. "Especially if we need to cath him."

ER nurses were definitely more proficient than psychiatry floor nurses when it came to hands-on procedural matters, just as emergency medicine doctors were compared to psychiatrists.

"Okay," my supervisor relented, but was clearly frustrated.

When the test came back within a half hour, the results screamed "urine infection." Instead of changing the doses of his antipsychotic medications, we kept him on his outpatient regimen and started him on an antibiotic to treat his infection. Within a few days, he improved to his baseline, still with signs of psychotic thinking present, but functional enough to return to his group home. I wasn't sure we would have obtained this sample on the psych unit in such a timely fashion. Untreated, his infection might have worsened to a level that required more aggressive medication treatment.

I brought these experiences with me—stories of disconnects between medicine and psychiatry—as I took in what Sanjeev, the surgeon, told me about Lennie. It sounded as if, in focusing exclusively on his head, several doctors might have overlooked what was going on down near his toes.

LENNIE DIDN'T WANT TO SEE ME. FOR SOME PATIENTS ON THE general hospital wards, talking with a psychiatric consultant offered hope that someone understood their struggles. For others, it signaled failure, that the medical team had given up on them. A third cohort approached us with fear and disdain. That's where Lennie landed.

"I don't need to go back to the crazy ward," he said to me after I introduced myself. "They sure as hell didn't help me."

He stared at what remained of his left leg, bandaged below the knee. I'd gone out of my way to avoid looking at his leg, but why? I'd been a doctor for over two years and a medical student before that; certainly, I'd seen my share of gruesome scenes. Something about the situation felt volatile, though, and I didn't want to make it even worse.

"The focus now is on your recovery from surgery," I said. "I'm here because your surgeons just want to make sure that you're safe."

"You mean like I'm gonna hurt myself or someone else?" he asked incredulously.

"Well, yes, I need to check in on those things," I stammered, "but also—"

Lennie cut me off, waving his hands, his skin worn and leathery like an old football. With his fleshy face, full gray beard, and thick neck, he could have been a convincing black Santa Claus in another life. But our present circumstances offered no space to indulge childhood fantasies.

"There's no way I would hurt myself," he fumed. "I wouldn't give those doctors and nurses at the other hospitals that kind of satisfaction. And as far as hurting someone else, how am I supposed to do that from here on one fucking leg?"

Lennie's words stung like a slap across my mouth. Technically, I could have checked off the "safety assessment" box that he wasn't suicidal or homicidal, and just gone through the motions from there. I'd done that before with some patients who complained about their medical care, knowing that often it was easier for them to blame their doctors than to accept their conditions.

But the sight of him without part of his leg somehow made me take his concerns of possible malpractice more seriously. I couldn't say that to him, though, since it would have been improper to speculate about medical colleagues I didn't even know on a situation I'd only entered after everything was over. In fact, I was unsure what to say at all. Platitudes that I was "sorry" or that "I couldn't imagine how hard this was" seemed fake and hollow.

Thankfully, Lennie continued, his voice calmer. "Look man, the Indian doctor told me I was going to have to talk to a shrink since I came from a mental ward at the other hospital. And I saw how the nurse got all scared when I told her how I felt about that place. You know, they always fear the 'angry black man,' even if he's a damn cripple."

Lennie laughed as he looked at his leg stump. I grimaced. I thought he was going to start crying or yelling, but he kept laughing.

"Ain't that some ironic shit?" he continued.

I'd seen doctors in these situations, when patients faced terrible news, start muttering awkwardly about the various ways the medical team could make things better. After all, nearly all doctors are motivated to help people, to fix their problems. There is perhaps nothing worse, in their eyes, than feeling powerless over suffering.

Instead of going down that rambling path, I kept quiet as Lennie stopped laughing. It wasn't that I knew how to skillfully employ silence for therapeutic benefit. Rather, I still didn't know what to say.

Lennie scanned me. "You're a big black dude. You must have gotten some of that. People being scared of you and all."

"Sure," I said simply. "No doubt about it. Even around here."

"I'm not surprised," Lennie replied. "I'm sure you have lots of stories."

Indeed, I could have recounted all sorts of experiences. Like the time a clerk on a medical ward almost called security when I entered the work area, assuming I was an intrusive family member rather than a doctor. Or when I got pulled from a patient's care because the man told my team that I looked just like someone who'd mugged him years earlier. But whatever obstacles I'd faced, I was still a doctor with a promising future. The good far outweighed the bad. Any details I might offer to him would pale in comparison to his life. He'd just lost his foot and part of his leg.

I hadn't said much, but the little I had seemed to soften the wall Lennie had put up to protect himself. I sensed an opening to connect with him.

"You mentioned a minute ago being admitted to the psych ward. From the records, it looks like you sought out help. Can you tell me a little about what led you to doing that?"

Lennie sighed as he pushed his torso deep into the mattress and repositioned his good leg. The short story was one I'd heard variations of many times before and since. In a span of two years, he'd gotten divorced, lost his job, and started drinking large amounts of alcohol. He gained thirty pounds, and his physical health declined.

"Did you see a mental health provider during this time?" I asked.

He told me his primary doctor gave him an antidepressant drug, but he didn't like the way it made him feel, sort of like he was in slow motion. She tried to refer him to a psychologist or psychiatrist, but none were available, especially after he'd lost his health insurance. At this point in training, I was just beginning to understand how difficult it was for people to get outpatient mental health treatment, psychotherapy especially, unless they could afford $200 visits for semiweekly sessions. Primary care doctors tried to fill much of this gap, mostly by prescribing pills.

Things continued to worsen for Lennie until the prior week, when he reached his low point. "I was driving on the road," he said, "thinking about how much of a failure my life was, and as I came up on this bridge, one lane each way, I got this thought in my head, you know, to just drive into the water below."

I'd heard patients recount some version of "driving into a tree" or "driving off a cliff" or "driving into a lake" nearly a dozen times in my year-plus of psychiatry training then. These stories always unnerved me, because, in contrast, I perpetually feared losing control of my car on a slippery roadway in treacherous conditions. I hated driving over bridges and through mountains, and periodically had nightmares of plunging to my death. I wondered if life could ever take me to a place where my mind harbored thoughts of self-destruction.

Lennie stared intensely at the wall behind me. It seemed he was putting himself back at the scene. During my stints at the VA hospital, I'd been cautioned not to push veterans too hard to recount their combat traumas overseas, or, in the case of far too many women I'd seen, their exposure to sexual assault. How much they revealed needed to be on their terms, I'd been told, not mine. Instinctively, I wanted to take the conversation in a different direction, to something less gloomy, the way most people would when faced with a person in despair. Instead, I kept quiet. And Lennie continued his story.

"I started to veer off right before the bridge," he began, "but then I swerved back and almost ran into a car coming from the other direction. We both slammed on our brakes. It was real close. That car had a mom with her two kids. That spooked me real bad, and I decided to take myself to the hospital."

When Lennie arrived at the hospital, he wasn't legally drunk, but he did have alcohol in his system. While I'd always been far more sympathetic to victims than offenders when it came to breaking the law, my time in psychiatry had begun to make me less judgmental about human fallibility. Lennie seemed genuinely contrite, and thankfully, the mom and children had not been physically injured.

Lennie's primary care doctor had diagnosed him with diabetes the last time he'd seen her, but he missed his follow-up appointment and stopped the medicine she'd given him to control his blood sugar right after he discarded the one she prescribed for his depression. When he got to the emergency room, he noticed his left foot ached. It had felt numb a few days earlier. The doctors there ordered an X-ray.

"They said it wasn't broken," Lennie said. "But none of them actually looked at my foot, you know, to examine it or nothing. None of them doctors did."

I'd had several busy nights in crowded hospitals where I'd done cursory physical exams. Sometimes the patient was agitated and uncooperative; other times I was pulled in too many directions and couldn't do more; and always, it seemed, I was brutally tired. Lennie had gone to a small, local hospital where he'd been triaged as a "psych case," and since that hospital didn't have a psychiatric unit, their overriding focus was to send him somewhere that did. I knew that mindset well. I hoped that I hadn't missed something on one of my long shifts that later caused a patient real harm.

Things didn't change when Lennie got to the psychiatric hospital. He arrived on a Friday afternoon, just as the regular weekday crew was leaving. An older psychiatrist interviewed him but didn't look at his feet, because a physical exam wasn't needed since Lennie had been "medically cleared" by the referring emergency room. Within an hour, he was under the covers in his assigned bed, where he remained for the rest of that day and most of Saturday morning. Nurses opened the door every fifteen minutes to make sure he was still alive, but otherwise left him alone. When he got up to use the bathroom around lunchtime, his foot still hurt, now more intensely.

"It felt like someone stuck me with a knife," he told me.

The nurse called the doctor, who ordered medication that put him to sleep. When he woke up several hours later, the stabbing pain was gone; now, his foot felt numb. The next morning, Sunday, he looked at his left foot and saw that it was swollen and had turned a bluish color. He could barely move his toes. He demanded that a doctor come to see him and look at his foot. A thirtysomething doctor arrived a short while later.

"She said, 'Oh my God,'" Lennie stated, recounting the scene to me. "That's what she said when she saw my foot. I'll never forget the way she said that and the look on her face. Never. That girl was white as a damn ghost."

The psych hospital transferred him by ambulance to our facility, where he was admitted to our surgery team. Suddenly, everyone was interested in his foot. They poked and prodded him as they examined every aspect of his lower body from groin to toe. They ordered various radiology and other imaging tests to measure blood flow throughout his legs.

He'd never seen doctors so eager to treat him. But it was too late. By day's end, the surgeons delivered the news that he needed an amputation to spare what was left.

"And now here I am," Lennie said as he looked down at his leg stump again, only this time he wasn't laughing at all.

My pager beeped. It was my coresident letting me know he was back at the hospital.

"You need to get that?" Lennie asked.

I shook my head. I realized that I'd made a major mistake in terms of bedside interviewing. Flustered at first by his anger and then later captivated by his story, I'd been standing up the entire time, towering over a man who'd lost part of his leg. One of the core lessons of medicine (psychiatry included) was to try to put the patient at ease, to meet them at their level whenever possible. Sitting down beside them was Doctoring 101.

"Can I have a seat?" I asked, pointing to the nearby cloth chair.

"Sure."

In truth, there was no "medical" reason for me to stay. I'd gotten enough information to complete my psychiatric consultation. I would recommend that the surgeons continue the antidepressant medication Lennie started at the psychiatric hospital. Our team would check on Lennie each day he remained in the hospital and arrange for him to continue mental health treatment once he left. On a surface level, it was that simple. Besides, my workload was piling up; I had other patients that I needed to see. But as I took in everything I'd learned about Lennie, it seemed that, first and foremost, the people who'd seen him hadn't really listened to him and gotten past the surface labels. Depression. Alcohol use. Psych patient. I'd been guilty of that narrow-minded approach with other patients, so in that moment, I tried to make up for my own failures as well as those of the doctors who'd seen him so far.

"Where did you grow up?" I asked.

Lennie smiled for the first time. "DC," he said. "Good old Chocolate City."

In the late 1950s, Washington, DC, became the first majority-black large city in the United States; by the 1970s, over 70 percent of its residents identified as black, thus the moniker.

I told Lennie that I grew up ten minutes away in Maryland. Most Sundays, I drove into the city with my mom to attend church and to visit my grandmother afterward. Many aunts, uncles, and cousins lived there too.

Lennie's smile grew wider. "I knew you seemed all right," he said.

He talked about how much he loved football and track growing up, and recounted his competitions with peers who went on to success in college and beyond. Lennie started out as a college athlete himself, but said he got "caught up with the wrong crowd" and soon lost his desire to be a student or an athlete. He left school midway through his second year.

"Biggest mistake of my life," he told me.

Lennie eventually went into the navy, got married, and moved to North Carolina, where he found steady work as a truck driver.

"Things were going good," he said wistfully.

Lennie didn't mention how his life began to detour (including an arrest for a drug charge that I later learned about), and I didn't feel there was any use in my probing further about his failed marriage, as it didn't matter to our conversation in the moment. He circled back to sports, asking about my time playing basketball in high school and college. He started smiling again.

We probably could have kept talking for much longer, but my pager beeped again.

"Looks like you've got other places to be, Doc," he said. "Other people to see. I do appreciate you talkin' with me, though."

"It's been nice talking with you too," I said. "I loved growing up in the DC area too."

"As for why you came to see me," he said, his expression turning solemn again, "nothing's gonna bring my leg back, but I'll be okay. I'm gonna do my therapy and get one of those prosthetic limbs. And then I'm gonna sue those bastards. That'll be my revenge."

Lennie's final words stayed with me as I saw other patients, and were fresh in my mind when I spoke with Sanjeev, the surgery resident, a few hours later. I told him that Lennie posed no immediate safety risks and that we'd follow him daily while he was in the hospital.

"Sounds good to me," Sanjeev said. "That's what I hoped. The last thing this guy needed was to be interrogated by police on post-op day one."

I thought back to our initial conversation where Sanjeev said he'd persuaded his supervisor to call me instead of the police. Why had that doctor's first impulse been to contact law enforcement? I had some ideas, but I'd never be able to prove any of them.

"That would have been absolutely awful," I said. "I'm glad I was able to help."

"I feel terrible for the guy," Sanjeev said. "He really caught a bad break."

Surgeons often have a reputation for being arrogant and callous, unconcerned with their patients outside of the operating room. While some lived down to that stereotype, many others, such as Sanjeev, were just the opposite.

"So do you think," I began, "that it was really a medical oversight, like he's describing it to us, which was the cause of him needing the amputation?"

Medical oversight was a euphemism for something I couldn't bring myself to say. This phrasing made it seem as if something benign might have occurred, like a very brief delay in prescribing a medication or in ordering a routine blood test. But what Lennie alleged was more appropriately called *medical malpractice*. This term, to my ears, implied something egregious occurred and that this negligence led to his terrible outcome.

"It's definitely possible," Sanjeev said. "My attending thinks someone dropped the ball. But it might be hard to prove that they should have caught the problem sooner. Or that they missed something obvious when he was in the ER, or when he came to the psych ward."

Sanjeev told me that the pre-templated records from the ER indicated a normal lower-extremity exam. Whether the doctors actually examined his foot, or whether they did not, as we suspected, would be unknown based on his chart. At best, they had done their jobs, and Lennie, racked with severe depression, simply didn't recall this. At worst, they'd covered their asses by checking off something that they hadn't actually done.

"But if a screwup from their end did cause this," Sanjeev continued, "it really reminds you of the stakes."

"For sure," I said as I recalled some of the many late-night cursory physicals I'd done.

Lennie came to the hospital ailing both in mind and body. But his psychiatric illness had seemingly made the doctors overlook his physical distress, or at least cut corners. The fact that he was a black man of limited financial means surely worsened his prospects for optimal care. I left the hospital late that evening determined to learn what options he had to redress the harm he'd suffered and vowing to do better for future patients.

IT TURNS OUT THAT MUCH OF WHAT DOCTORS HEAR ABOUT MEDICAL malpractice early in their training isn't true. Or at least that was so for me. In medical school, we didn't have a formal lecture or other cohesive overview of the subject. Instead, we learned about it in piecemeal fashion from supervisors at our various clinical sites. I heard surgeons describe patients with "unrealistic expectations," internists who feared "missing a zebra," and obstetricians lamenting that they could be sued until their patients turned eighteen.

Implied across specialties was the idea that doctors were subject to frivolous lawsuits by an increasingly ungrateful public who were seeking lottery-like jury verdicts, egged on by unscrupulous ambulance-chasing lawyers whose earnings far exceeded our own. In this narrative, doctors found themselves forced to practice "defensive medicine," ordering unneeded CT scans, biopsies, and medicines. I had no reason to question its truth.

But in the waning months of medical school, I stumbled upon a mid-afternoon presentation where the speaker challenged everything I had informally learned over the years. I'd initially been attracted to the warm food outside the lecture hall, yet felt a sense of obligation to at least peek inside. To my surprise, I was immediately engaged. The professor, an emergency medicine physician who also had an MBA, vividly described a real-life case involving a woman who ended up with a "bad clinical outcome" related to a surgical procedure. In contrast to the perception that she would walk away with millions, she ended up with nothing as the jury ruled for the doctors. This outcome highlighted his first point: that most juries sided with doctors over plaintiffs in malpractice verdicts. He then explained how the overwhelming majority of claims never made it to a jury verdict; they were either settled or dismissed.

While the doctor perspective I'd been indoctrinated to embrace saw malpractice as a force that threatened our survival as physicians, this speaker charged us to consider the patient perspective and to advocate for malpractice reform in such a way that we might do better by our patients as a whole without unduly blaming an individual doctor or group of doctors.

That central message floated through my mind as I contemplated Lennie's situation. It seemed unclear whether he would actually be able to prove in a court of law that the physicians at the two other hospitals had committed genuine malpractice. The doctors' notes from our hospital were worded so as not to directly impugn their colleagues elsewhere, probably at least in part because they didn't want someone to later critically judge them. But Lennie had walked into the hospital on his own two feet and would limp away without a foot and part of his leg. Maybe those hospitals would give a cash settlement. Or nothing.

But another thought circulated in my head. Could Lennie's amputation have been prevented? Would doctors more fully attuned to both physical and mental health have minimized the damage? A few days after meeting Lennie, I worked a Friday night shift in the ER, where a doctor showed me what integrated care from head to toe could look like.

THE YOUNG WOMAN STARED AT ME. AND KEPT STARING. HER DEEP-SET eyes unnerved me.

"Are you an African prince?" Jade asked. "We could have lots of children together. They would grow up to be princes and princesses too."

I looked at the nursing assistant behind me, who struggled to suppress her smile.

"No, I'm a doctor," I said gently. "And you're at the hospital. In the emergency room."

I did not mention that I was a psychiatrist, not knowing how she'd respond, since her records indicated she'd never seen a mental health professional.

"Oh," she said blankly. "I haven't been feeling great. But I think I'm getting better."

I looked down at the nursing triage form. It started off: "Twenty-two-year-old black female with recent-onset psychosis." The note then indicated that she'd been brought by her father for a one-week history of increasingly bizarre behavior that included repetitively mumbling to herself, laughing inappropriately, cursing profusely, and sleeping only two or three hours each night. She'd missed a week of work and was told she needed to "get well" before she could return.

"What has been bothering you?" I asked.

"Do you like to take ice baths?" she replied. "They make my hands feel real good. Can I touch your hands?"

The rest of the interview confirmed that her thinking and speech patterns weren't logical, at least not to me or her family. It was Friday evening, and I tried to imagine Jade, dressed in stylish clothes and jewelry, hanging out with work friends at a bar decompressing from a busy week. Instead, she'd been placed in faded purple hospital scrubs with no jewelry allowed in the locked mental health unit.

After a few minutes, Jade's playful mood abruptly vanished and she became upset with the nursing assistant, throwing f-bombs in her direction for unclear reasons. We calmly exited the room, leaving Jade alone in the locked patient area.

"Sorry about that," I said to the nursing aide.

The triage nurse had taken Jade's vital signs on arrival: her heart rate, pulse, and oxygen saturation were within the normal range. She didn't have a fever. The nurse had drawn blood for the standard set of labs and gotten a urine sample from Jade right before I began my interview. Assuming those results checked out fine, we'd send her upstairs to the psychiatric unit, or to another psychiatric hospital if no beds were available on ours.

As I headed to my workroom space down the hall, I saw Dr. Landis, the lead emergency physician on the medical wing, approach. He was midthirties and still single, and enjoyed the freedom that brought. We'd crossed paths at the campus gym a few times, and he'd encouraged me to start playing tennis instead of simply watching it on TV. After a few frustrating outings, the game was steadily growing on me.

"You here to see our patient?" I asked him.

Each patient in the psychiatric wing needed to be seen and examined by an ER physician for what we called *medical clearance*, to ensure that the patient didn't have some life-threatening medical issue needing attention. Any medical needs short of that, they left to us in psychiatry to manage. Usually, this duty to "clear" our patients fell to one of the emergency medicine residents, but this time Dr. Landis came personally to do the initial assessment.

"We're getting slammed on the other side," he explained to me, "so I figured I'd knock this one out quickly."

"Sure," I said. "Vitals look good. We're waiting on labs."

"The nurse mentioned something about her hands being a little swollen?"

I looked at him blankly, like an unprepared student who'd been called on in class. Then I looked down at the triage nurse entry I'd printed. The bulk of her note talked about Jade's psychiatric symptoms. Buried in the middle, though, it did mention that she'd had some pain in her fingers and wrists.

"I didn't notice anything," I said. "I was going to go back later and examine her depending upon where she ends up."

As psychiatrists working in the emergency department, we were expected to do physical exams for patients we admitted upstairs to our unit. But for those we sent elsewhere, we could rely on the ER physician evaluation. I didn't fully understand the logic behind these rules but felt no need to challenge them by doing extra work.

"You have time now?" he asked. "To go take a look?"

"Y-yes," I stammered.

Jade looked puzzled by the presence of two white-coated doctors. Many times, I wondered how people in the midst of psychosis perceived me and their surroundings. Did I look like a "normal" person trying to help them through a difficult time, or did our surroundings make them think I was a devious researcher seeking to torture them? Thankfully, Jade, while clearly confused, didn't seem distressed.

"Is this your friend?" she asked me as she looked at Dr. Landis. "He's cute too. Is he from Sweden?"

Dr. Landis pleasantly introduced himself and explained his role as a lead physician in the emergency department.

"That's right," Jade said in a moment of clarity. "I'm in a hospital."

"Can I look at your hands?" Dr. Landis asked.

On close inspection, some of the joints in her fingers were a little swollen. Dr. Landis then used a penlight to examine the skin on her arms and neck area.

"Those could be rashes," he said, pointing to a few small areas of paler discoloration.

"Is everything okay?" Jade asked.

"Yes," Dr. Landis replied. "We're just giving you a good checkup."

"Good," she replied. "I need one. Everyone needs one. Doctors too."

"You had any fevers recently?" Dr. Landis asked, calmly refocusing her.

"Cold baths help," she said. "The cold feels good."

"Nice to meet you," Dr. Landis said after asking a few other questions. "Dr. Tweedy and I are going to step outside. We'll come back and talk to you later."

By the time we left the workstation, I'd pieced together Dr. Landis's clinical thinking. Fever, rash, and joint swelling in a young black woman. While this cluster of information could mean many things, we'd all been taught to focus on one diagnosis in particular.

"So you're thinking lupus?" I asked him.

Lupus is an autoimmune disease, meaning it's a disease in which the immune system attacks the body's own tissues. Ninety percent of cases occur in women, developing between the teenage years and early thirties. While it affects all racial groups, in the US, black women are about three times more likely than white women to be diagnosed with lupus, making it a classic case of the seemingly many diseases "more common in blacks than in whites," a disturbing refrain I heard so often throughout medical training.

"It's certainly possible," he said. "We'll need to get lab work. I'll put in those orders."

Good clinical work, for sure, I thought, but the kind that a rheumatologist or primary care doctor could do in an outpatient office. We were in the psychiatric wing of the emergency unit. Why was he chasing down a diagnosis seemingly irrelevant to what had brought her there? I was about to say as much when it all suddenly clicked.

"Neuropsychiatric lupus!" I exclaimed. "Is that what you're thinking?"

The women I'd seen with serious lupus complications had heart, kidney, and lung problems. Some had depression and anxiety too, although it was hard to know if that was the biological effect of the disease itself or a reaction to its many disabling features. I'd read in textbooks that lupus could cause mania or psychosis, but had never seen that.

Dr. Landis nodded. "Given that possibility, I think we need to admit her to Medicine over the weekend and transfer her to the Med-Psych team on Monday."

"Oh . . . okay," I said. "That makes sense."

The change of plans stunned me. Assuming her urine drug screen wasn't positive for psychoactive drugs, such as cocaine, PCP, or marijuana, I'd been anticipating that Jade would be admitted to an inpatient psychiatric unit to treat her new-onset psychosis with an antipsychotic drug like risperidone. That's what we did most of the time. Default mode. Instead, we were now talking about additional blood tests and potentially using entirely different types of drugs: corticosteroids, hydroxychloroquine, and other immune suppressants.

"I could be totally wrong, and this could just be schizophrenia," he said. "But if there's any chance this is lupus or some other autoimmune disorder, we need to rule that out. I'll call the Medicine team, and we'll go from there."

We spent the next minute or two talking about tennis before Dr. Landis headed back to the medical wing. After reviewing her electronic chart for lab test results, I went out to the emergency department waiting area to update Jade's father on her status. He was middle-aged, balding on top, with coarse hands that looked as if he'd spent much of his life doing physical labor. He stood anxiously as I approached and introduced myself.

"Hello, Doctor," he said to me. "How is Jade?"

I explained to him that although she had been sent to us for delusional thinking and behaviors, our medical evaluation suggested that she needed additional studies to rule out potential medical causes for her mental status changes. I left out the part about me missing those possible clinical clues and Dr. Landis finding them.

"You mean drugs?" he asked.

Her urine drug screen, which I'd just reviewed, hadn't detected any drugs. But it didn't test all possibilities. The list of mind-altering substances was seemingly limitless.

"Does she have a history of drug use? Anything you could point to recently?"

"Not that we know of," he answered. "Not now or in the past."

"Is she taking any prescription pills or supplements or vitamins?" I asked.

He shook his head. "We thought maybe she had started smoking weed or something. Me and my wife went through her bathroom, her purse, under her bed, everywhere. We didn't find nothing. Just an old bottle of Motrin and some vitamin C pills."

Neither of which were the culprits. I tried to picture the scene at their home, this man and his wife turning over their daughter's possessions like officers executing a search warrant, scouring through every aspect of her life for any clue that might yield evidence of what had taken over her mind.

"We're actually thinking more along the lines of a medical condition—something happening on its own—as the cause for her mental changes," I said to him.

He looked confused. "Like what?"

There are many medical problems that can cause psychosis, ranging from a dangerously overactive thyroid gland, to a variety of metabolic deficiencies that prevent the body from clearing toxins, to actual brain injury or infection.

"I don't want to get ahead of things," I said, "but our plan is to test her for lupus."

Lupus doesn't have a specific diagnostic test. Instead the diagnosis relies on a checklist, where a certain number of findings need to be present from a larger list. This is similar to the way psychiatrists go about diagnosing depression, bipolar disorder, or PTSD. Only no one contests its legitimacy the way some do psychiatric diagnoses.

"I've heard of that," he said as he took in this update, his voice growing quieter. "Saw something on TV about it not too long ago. So you think that could explain what's been happening to her . . . to her . . . mind?"

"Possibly," I said.

His eyes widened. "And so you don't think she has s-schizo . . . ?"

Schizophrenia doesn't easily roll off the tongue. I'm not sure I could have pronounced it before my psychology class in college. But he knew what it meant: "crazy." Clearly, that label had been the unspoken thing he had feared the most.

"We're not sure," I said honestly. "Right now, I just wanted to make sure you knew where things stood. She's going upstairs to the medical floor tonight. Someone from their team will get in touch with you once she's settled up there."

"So she's not going to the psycho ward?" he asked even more softly, almost in a whisper, his eyes scanning the area to see if anyone might hear us.

"At least not for now," I said. "But there'll be some psychiatrists who will see her when she's upstairs on the medical ward."

Jade's dad sighed, seemingly in relief. "Thank you so much, Doctor."

What I'd seen of lupus from patients over the years hadn't been pretty. It affected multiple organ systems in much the same way as diabetes. I suspected Jade's dad didn't really understand the trajectory of lupus. But maybe even if he had, the idea of a "physical" condition, whatever it might bring, somehow still seemed a lot better than schizophrenia or bipolar disorder. In the eyes of many patients and family members I'd met over the years, there was nothing worse than a psychiatric illness.

I soon got busy with other patients for the rest of my shift as Friday night turned into Saturday morning. Jade went upstairs to the medical ward shortly after midnight. When I returned to the hospital that Monday, I tracked down Dr. Bales, a Med-Psych physician, to find out what happened to Jade. Dr. Bales had just left a patient room, her shoes making a distinct clicking with each step on the hospital tile.

"Did you get a transfer this morning from the Gen Med team that came through the ER on Friday night / Saturday morning?" I asked her after we'd exchanged pleasantries.

"Sure," she said. "Looks like lupus psychosis. That was a good catch you all made downstairs to get her sent up here to a medicine floor."

"Dr. Landis," I replied. "He's sharp. I've got to give him all the credit."

"Oh yeah, he's really good," she agreed. "He would have made a great internist."

Around the hospital, *internists*, doctors trained in general internal medicine and its various subspecialties, were commonly seen as the keenest physicians in terms of making complicated diagnoses. Dr. Bales, as a Med-Psych physician, was trained in both internal medicine and psychiatry.

"Sometimes ER docs get a bad rap," she continued, "but it's not easy work they do. And there are some gems like him."

"What's your plan for her?" I asked.

Dr. Bales deftly explained the ongoing evaluation and initial treatments for suspected lupus while remaining fully attentive to the psychiatric aspects of Jade's case. Given that I'd spent a year in both general medicine and psychiatry at that point, I was impressed with her ability to integrate her knowledge of both fields. Then again, her training had made her ideally suited for this. Duke had operated a Med-Psych program for more than a decade, and over the years, these doctors had increasingly taken over much of the hospital's emergency-level psychiatric care, where general medicine and psychiatry were most likely to intersect.

"You know it's not too late for you to join us," Dr. Bales said with a full smile. "We'd love to have you."

When I began thinking about leaving the general medicine residency program and switching into psychiatry, I seriously considered joining the Med-Psych program. But completing two residencies simultaneously felt like too much for where I was at the moment, as it would have added more time to my training years before I could become a full-fledged doctor. Besides, my goal in starting general medicine had been to eventually work as a cardiologist, and the years needed to become a cardiologist-psychiatrist—a decade—were far more than I could manage, financially, physically, or emotionally. So I gave up the dream of becoming an expert in the inner workings of the heart for the murkier task of trying to understand the mind.

"Maybe in another life," I said jokingly. "Psychiatry alone is excitement enough."

"It's definitely not boring," Dr. Bales said. "That's for sure."

Jade's case reaffirmed what had attracted me to psychiatry in the first place, vividly showing how the mind and body could not be neatly divided from each other. Certainly not in the way it was done by insurance companies, medical schools, and in what I heard in everyday conversation with friends and strangers outside the health care world. Being a good internist, surgeon, or ER doctor required understanding the emotional dimensions of health; likewise, a good psychiatrist needed to avoid becoming too detached from their patients' physical well-being. Watching Dr. Landis and Dr. Bales in action highlighted what medicine, and psychiatry, could look like at their best.

Seeing the exemplary care that Jade received brought my thoughts back to Lennie. His immediate postamputation recovery proceeded smoothly, and he was transferred to a skilled nursing facility to begin the next steps: a program of more rigorous physical therapy and starting the process of adapting to his future life with a prosthetic limb. We would never cross paths again, but he would remain a part of me. From what I could piece together, the doctors he'd seen at his local emergency room were no Dr. Landis, nor were the psychiatrists at the local psychiatric hospital on par with Dr. Bales. But maybe my judgment was too harsh, and the real problem for these doctors was the settings in which they worked. Were the procedures of patient care—too many patients and too few staff—a recipe for medical error, no matter how competent or well-intentioned the physicians and nurses?

I'd never know the answer, but I couldn't help thinking that if Lennie had encountered Dr. Landis and Dr. Bales, there would have been no need for lawyers or hospital risk managers or malpractice insurers, because he would still have had both of his legs, fully intact.

PART III

CENTERING

7

LOST AND FOUND

IT ALL STARTED WITH A CAR RIDE. ON A WARM, LATE-WINTER MORNING, Earl, a seventy-nine-year-old retired truck driver, told his wife that he was going to the local hardware store to buy a new water sprinkler for their lawn. He liked working with his hands, and spent most mornings doing outdoor projects on their rural one-acre property. Shortly after 9:00 A.M., he got behind the wheel of his Ford pickup truck, as he'd done countless times before to run errands. Only on this day, he never made it to his destination.

After an hour, his wife, Sally, started to worry. She called his cell phone, but heard it ring in the other room; once again, he'd left it at home, probably on purpose, she thought. She waited another half hour before calling April, her older daughter, who lived ten minutes away. April sped to the hardware store. The manager, who knew Earl, said that he hadn't come by that morning. April then raced to the local Walmart, but couldn't find any sign of her dad. Desperate, she drove to other common places her father went: the grocery store, the pharmacy, the local bank. Still no signs of him. Fearing the worst, by 11:30 A.M., she called the police.

I shared this story and its aftermath with Dr. Davenport, the senior psychiatrist who supervised the outpatient resident clinic where I worked Wednesday afternoons. I'd just seen Earl and his family, and told them that I'd call them after I had the chance to discuss his case with my supervisor.

"So what are your thoughts?" Dr. Davenport asked me.

We sat in his spacious corner office, adorned with bookshelves full of tomes about psychiatry, psychology, neurology, and general medicine.

"This seems like straightforward dementia," I said. "Probably Alzheimer's in the early to middle stages. So I'm thinking we should probably transfer him to a neurology clinic."

Dr. Davenport loosened his necktie. His thinning hair was well-groomed and his face clean-shaven. He eschewed glasses in favor of contacts.

"What are you thinking they could offer him that we couldn't?" he asked me.

Neurologists focus on diseases of the brain and its tentacles, such as strokes, multiple sclerosis, ALS, and Parkinson's, that commonly have physical manifestations, in contrast to the psychiatrists' emphasis on disturbances in thought, mood, and emotion that usually do not result in abnormal neurological findings. Dementia, a disease of the brain whose primary impact is behavioral rather than physical, straddles both disciplines.

A few weeks had passed since the incident in question, and Earl had seen emergency medicine doctors as well as his primary care physician. He'd gone through various blood and radiology tests that might have offered alternative diagnoses. Dementia was at the top of everyone's list of potential explanations. But these doctors, perhaps because of how hopeless the condition seemed, had been reluctant to tell this directly to the family.

"Maybe the neurologists could get him into a clinical study," I said. "To try something that might slow the course of his disease."

Dr. Davenport looked at me with curiosity, as if my response surprised him. "We have folks in our department who are doing dementia-related studies as well."

"So you think we should send him to geriatric psych instead?" I asked.

"We could. Did the family indicate that they were interested in a clinical study?"

"No," I started, then stopped as I tried to self-correct. "I didn't ask them specifically. They mainly just wanted a tangible diagnosis and information on what the next steps are."

Dr. Davenport pushed his chair back from his desk to give himself enough room to cross his legs, with his right foot resting on his left knee.

"We can definitely talk to them about whether he meets inclusion criteria for any ongoing studies," he said. "But I think we're getting ahead of ourselves a bit. For starters, I'm getting the sense that this patient is making you uncomfortable, and that you want to discard him."

Instinctively, I felt defensive. It seemed in that moment as if he were trying to psychoanalyze me in classic psychiatrist fashion. I'd reviewed patient cases with Dr. Davenport at least a half dozen times before, and, while he was always thorough, he'd never come across so heavy-handedly.

In response to his implication that I wanted to "hot potato" Earl onto someone else, I countered with a response that I thought was unassailable in its noble intentions.

"Well, as we all know," I began, "dementia is a very bad disease. So I figure we should be as aggressive as possible from the outset in trying to slow its course and maybe make it be not so severe in the end. That's how I'm seeing it."

I'd fallen back on standard medical thinking. People come to us in distress, and our goal is to fix the problem or, when that's not possible, to at least make it less problematic. While psychiatric treatments are more mystical than surgery or antibiotics, they help many people. But there is no magic bullet to treat dementia. Nothing even close.

"I can understand how a patient like this would be hard to see," Dr. Davenport replied, as if he had listened to my inner dialogue. "It's unsettling to be confronted with someone we can't do much to help. Sometimes we blame the patient and get angry at them. In a case like this where we can't do that, it's easier to avoid them altogether."

I knew what he meant, and agreed that it made sense. Still, I didn't know how to respond, so I reverted back to medical-doctor mode.

"We can start him on donepezil," I offered. "But I'd want to make sure that being on it is not an exclusion criteria for a clinical study. That's another reason to give them more information on potential studies sooner rather than later."

Donepezil belonged to a class of drugs that came on the market in the 1990s, marketed to improve cognitive function in the earlier stages of dementia. A newer drug, one that worked through a different mechanism, had recently been released too.

"These are things to discuss with the patient and his family," Dr. Davenport replied. "In my experience, it's also important for everyone to start thinking about daily-life things. For instance, are they on the same page about him not driving?"

"They're working on that," I said, recalling his insistence on not stopping altogether. "He's driven a few times with his wife in the car with him."

Dr. Davenport winced. "You can send a note to DMV for them to schedule a driving assessment. Hopefully, the family can work this out on their own. What about finances?"

"I'm not sure," I replied.

"That's important to sort out," Dr. Davenport said. "One time I saw a patient who spent a big part of his and his wife's joint retirement account by buying a high-end Mercedes that in the end he couldn't drive. I hope they got most of their money back, but I'm not sure."

I'd never asked a patient about their finances unless they'd brought it up for some specific reason, such as being unable to afford a prescription. Anything beyond that felt like something a medical social worker, not a physician, would need to consider.

"Do they have guns at home?"

"Yes," I said, feeling on more familiar footing as a doctor who dealt with suicidal patients frequently. "We talked about that, and they had already given them to his younger brother before all of this happened, because he'd stopped hunting a few years ago."

"Good. As you see, there is a lot more to this than drugs and clinical trials. Do you have any questions for me before you call them back?"

I jotted down notes on his recommendations. "No," I said, shaking my head.

He paused before speaking again. "They walked by here a few minutes before you came in. They seem like nice people. It's too bad dementia is such a terrible disease."

I saw the rest of my afternoon patients—all people I'd seen once or more previously, and all doing better—before calling Earl's number listed in the chart. His wife, Sally, answered.

"Thanks so much for calling like you said you would," she said.

It sounded like she'd been waiting for my call and that there had been occasions when medical people had disappointed her. I still hadn't fully embraced my identity as a doctor, the idea that, at any given time, I could be the most important person that a patient or family member heard from in a week, a month, a year, or perhaps longer. That felt like a lot more responsibility than I ever desired.

I went through the plan that I outlined with Dr. Davenport. Sally said she wanted to talk with her daughter about whether to pursue a clinical trial versus starting on one of the existing medications for dementia. We scheduled a follow-up visit in two weeks.

"Thanks again for calling me," she said. "We understand how busy you must be, and we promise to respect your time."

As I hung up the phone, Dr. Davenport's final words played in my head. They really did appear to be nice people. But based on the information we had, Earl had boarded the harrowing train toward becoming an old, confused person. And, although I'd never admitted it aloud, I didn't like seeing old, confused people. Neither did many of my colleagues in medicine.

DEMENTIA IS ONE OF THE MOST FEARED HEALTH CONDITIONS AMONG people over age fifty, and when younger people worry about becoming old, this disease is among their greatest concerns too. While there are several types of dementia, or neurocognitive disorders, that differ in various respects—Alzheimer's disease being the most common and well known—all ultimately impair the ability to think, communicate, remember, and carry out routine, everyday-life activities. Dementia robs us of what makes us distinctly human. It also takes an exacting toll on caregivers, who are mostly close family and friends.

Doctors struggle when providing care for these patients too. Traditional biomedical treatments are limited, and when we encounter people with dementia, especially during our formative training years, they are the ones who are often most sick, both cognitively and physically. Thus, while I didn't fully understand it at the time, one of my first lessons in the hospital as a medical student was to avoid having to treat confused elderly patients whenever possible.

This instruction didn't occur as part of formal lecture; in fact, we'd spent part of an afternoon months earlier in our Introduction to Medicine course learning about geriatrics, the specialty that focused on people over age sixty-five. A geriatric specialist (geriatrician) had given us a thirty-minute talk explaining how life expectancy in the US had steadily increased over the previous quarter century. His baby boomer generation was getting older at the same time that our Gen X cohort was having fewer kids. That meant there were going to be a lot more old people around, literally and proportionately, as time went on. He then highlighted the diversity of old people: some were vibrant into their eighties, while others had significant declines in their late sixties.

Next, we watched a narrated video accompanied by feel-good music that showed images of a hypothetical person at each stage of life from infancy to advanced age. The purpose was to illustrate the universal reality that unless one dies young, growing old was part of the inevitable cycle of life. But for a group of twentysomething medical students, the idea of being eighty-five one day seemed too far away to grasp; most of our parents were only in their fifties. Despite its good intentions, this single lecture that aimed to paint a sympathetic portrait on aging was no match for the reality that confronted me once I set foot in a hospital and saw how doctors interacted with certain elderly patients.

On the first day of my general internal medicine rotation several months later, our medical team discussed Mr. Wilcox, an elderly man on our patient roster. Chad, the second-year medical resident, looked at me.

"No, you don't want to see him," he said. "He's not a good teaching case. Not at all."

Jesse, the medical intern, felt similarly. "I agree," he said.

The three of us sat at a small conference table in a doctor workroom at the VA hospital. They were trying to determine which two patients to assign to me.

"Let's give you Barrett," Chad said, using last names only. "And Rice."

I looked down at the rounding sheet, which crammed pertinent medical information for the eight or nine patients from our team onto a single page. Barrett was in his midfifties and had come in for treatment of atrial fibrillation; Rice was a fortysomething with acute pancreatitis. Wilcox, the patient they'd told me to steer clear of, was a seventy-eight-year-old man with dementia who'd been admitted for pneumonia.

"Okay," I said, as facts about atrial fibrillation and pancreatitis rattled in my head.

A short while later, we walked onto the unit to see the people on our list. Three were in the "big room" that held eight patients, divided by curtains, military hospital–style; most of the others were in smaller rooms that held four patients each. Wilcox, in contrast, had a room all to himself. I asked Chad and Jesse why.

"Last time he was here four months ago, he was on contact precautions," Jesse said. "So we're just playing it safe until we get his sputum and blood cultures back."

Contact precautions meant he had an infection the hospital was worried medical staff could transmit between patients. We had to put on a disposable gown and gloves to enter his room, remove them as we left, and wash our hands vigorously at the nearby sink.

"And he's in another world," Chad said, as he twirled his index finger in small circles. "Thinks it's 1968 and Lyndon Johnson is president. The less folks around him, the better."

Chad and Jesse began to don their yellow gowns and latex gloves. I reached for these same items, but Chad stopped me.

"Don't worry about doing all that," he said. "You can stay outside and wait for us. Shouldn't be long. Like I said, he isn't a good teaching case. You'll have plenty of time to see someone with pneumonia who can actually tell you how they are feeling. You'll learn a lot more that way than with seeing this guy. We'll be quick."

Chad made it seem like he was protecting me. Interns and residents were real doctors who had to see everyone in the hospital, but medical students were there primarily to learn. In Chad's view, there wasn't any educational value in seeing an old guy with dementia.

For the next week, as patients on our service came and went, Mr. Wilcox remained in the same room. I never went inside.

One morning after we'd made rounds on our patient list, Patrice, the medical social worker assigned to our team, entered the workroom area. Her job was to coordinate discharge planning for those patients who required more than a prescription and a follow-up appointment with their primary care doctor. She handled placement in rehab facilities, home health care arrangements, and so forth. She had bad news. Or at least that's how it sounded to my team of overworked, stressed-out doctors.

"His daughter doesn't think she can take him back in with her in his present state," Patrice said.

Earlier that morning, I'd heard Chad tell Jesse that Mr. Wilcox was ready to be discharged. Patrice had just poured cold water on those plans.

"He came in with pneumonia, and we treated that," Chad said bluntly. "All his numbers are normal. We can't fix his dementia."

"She knows that," Patrice replied, "but she says he wasn't that unsteady on his feet before he came into the hospital. She doesn't think he'd be safe at home like he is now."

"I seriously doubt he was doing jumping jacks before he got admitted," Chad said.

Patrice took a slow, deep breath. She probably wanted to tell Chad that his sarcasm bordered on cruel, but decided it was best to keep things moving along.

"I suppose not," she said finally.

"Has PT been seeing him?" Chad asked Jesse.

Jesse clicked the mouse and scrolled through his chart. We had what was then a novel computerized record system at the VA hospital, one where notes from nurses, physical therapists, social workers, and occupational therapists were filed alongside physician entries. But as a medical student, I almost never opened these other notes, much less read through them. I'd already embraced the problematic ethos of the hospital hierarchy that anything of real value for a patient could be found in the doctors' writings.

"Yes," Jesse answered. "But it looks like his dementia is preventing him from following directions the way they need him to."

Chad squeezed his temples with his thumb and middle finger before he looked up. "Look, I realize it's a bad situation," he said to Patrice, appearing to walk back his earlier comments. "But we can't keep him in the hospital forever either. This isn't a nursing home."

"I know," Patrice agreed. "I'll see what kind of home health services he's eligible for. And I'll start looking for facilities to send him at the same time in case it doesn't work out."

Patrice briefly explained that Mr. Wilcox lived off a small social security check and that Medicaid offered limited placement options. At that point, medical school had focused mainly on physical diagnosis and drug or surgical treatments. I'd pushed aside the little I'd heard about health care systems and health insurance plans. Yet clearly, as she explained it to us, these seemingly mundane topics deeply affected our patients and their overall health.

Later that morning, we met with our attending, Dr. Markham. As we updated her on Mr. Wilcox, she immediately applied his situation to her own life.

"My dad had dementia too," she said, "but I'm really thankful he didn't drag on for too long before a heart attack took him away. Still, the last six months were very hard. Especially for my mom. But really for all of us. I just hope when her time comes, it will be even quicker. It will be hard no matter what, but I hope she doesn't suffer like this."

"My grandfather had ALS," Jesse said. "That was hard to watch too."

"Personally, if I could decide, I'd want to be pretty healthy until about eighty or so then lie down one night and not wake up the next morning,"

Chad added. "Short of that, I'd settle for a heart attack or aneurysm. It would be scary and painful, but it would be quick."

I didn't speak, but I had my own story. My grandmother had died almost two years earlier, during my second month of medical school. She'd suffered a stroke months before, one that caused severe physical and cognitive injuries. The last time I saw her, I'd gone with my mom to visit her at the rehabilitation facility where she'd been for a few weeks. She confused my mom—her eldest daughter—as being her sister. She didn't recognize me at all. We stayed for a half hour or so, enough time for my mom to talk to the nurses and doctors. As soon as we got into the car to drive back home, my mom started crying, something she rarely did. Weeks later, I was off to medical school, pushing aside the memory of that day.

In sharing her own family story and inviting us to mention ours, Dr. Markham had done something exceedingly rare in the emotionally detached, busy throes of hospital life: she'd gifted us the chance to reflect on how what we saw in the hospital applied to our own lives. What became evident is that we were all afraid of aging and death, both for those we loved and for our own future selves. And as I'd see during the remainder of that rotation, and years later during my internship, the easiest way to manage this fear was to avoid the issue altogether. That hidden or informal curriculum, as it is known, held far more influence over us future doctors than any single lecture or two could hope to provide.

Thus, when I met Earl and his family midway through my psychiatry residency, several years after that medical school experience, I had no reason to expect that my dealings with them would be any different from how it had been with other elderly patients I'd treated. But a life in medicine always comes with genuine surprises.

I KNEW A LOT ABOUT EARL BEFORE I EVER SPOKE TO HIM OR TO anyone else in his family. Or at least I thought so. In the half hour before his first appointment with me, I read through his medical chart, which included notes from an emergency department visit and from his primary care physician. His chart had lots of numbers and other clinical data: vital sign measurements, blood test results, CT scan findings, and physical exam summaries. His diagnosis of hypertension and the meds used to treat it came up several times. He didn't drink alcohol, smoke cigarettes, or use drugs. I'd even gotten a peek into his social life: he was a Raleigh native who'd previously been a truck driver for over thirty years. He'd been married to his high school sweetheart for over fifty years and had two grown daughters.

From a data standpoint, I knew more about Earl than I did my own brother, maybe even my parents. In reviewing his chart, I'd also learned enough, based on past experiences with other older confused patients, to feel unsettled. What could I offer him?

My stomach tensed when the front desk alerted me to his arrival. Moments later, Earl—accompanied by both an older woman and a younger one—stood at the entryway to a small shared office that I used on Wednesday afternoons.

"Could you get us an extra chair?" the older woman asked.

"Sure," I said as politely as I could muster. "Let me grab one from next door."

The square-shaped room had enough space for me to comfortably seat a patient in the cloth chair next to my work desk. Occasionally, a husband or wife might join us, in which case, they could sit in the wood chair that was mostly used for decoration or storage. For the first time in the six months I'd been working at this psychiatry resident clinic, I had to find room for three people: Earl, his wife, Sally, and their daughter April.

Earl smiled at me as I reentered the room and helped everyone get seated. Tall, lean, and with good posture, his physique could have passed for someone a decade younger. But his hair, all gray, and his wrinkled skin, which had patches of discoloration on his face and hands, were truer to his seventy-nine years.

"You're what kinda doctor again?" he asked me.

Sally and April shared a look equal parts embarrassment and frustration, as if they'd told him this information on the car ride to the clinic and again when they entered the building, but he'd already forgotten.

"Some general medicine," I said. "Mostly psychiatry though. I deal with mental health."

By this point, I was halfway done with my second year as a psychiatry resident, meaning I'd spent more time in this field than the year of general medicine I did previously. Still, I felt uncomfortable thinking of myself as a psychiatrist. Partly this was because I continued to spend most of my time in the hospital, pulling ER shifts, seeing consults on medical and surgical floors, and being the first contact for medical issues (such as chest pain or bloody diarrhea) that arose on the psychiatric units, which was not infrequent. In that way, I still felt like the white-coated doctor I'd set out to become when I started medical school. But I also knew that a lot of people—both within medicine and outside of it—didn't think of psychiatrists as medical doctors. Not real ones anyway. Given all the time I'd spent along the medical pathway, I didn't want to be seen that way.

"I'm not sure why I need to see you," Earl replied to me. "I have a regular doctor. And I feel mighty fine. I'm happy as a bird."

"Okay," I said. "That's good to hear."

Sally smiled and laughed uncomfortably. She wore a deep pink blouse, light gray pants, and crimson shoes, a color scheme that seemed to suggest she wanted to exude vitality. Her smooth white hair looked well-groomed.

"Earl's always been very positive," she said to me.

April, the daughter, frowned. In contrast to her mom, she seemed to prefer a lower-maintenance style: oversize athletic sweatshirt, blue jeans, and hiking boots.

"Have you read his chart?" she asked. "Do you know what happened last month?"

I told her that I had. About two hours after April called local police and provided them with her father's car and license plate information, officers in a neighboring county found Earl at a gas station terminal, his truck parked on the wrong side to fill up his tank. When they approached him, according to the medical notes, he told them that he'd gotten "turned around" but had figured out how to get back home and just needed some gas.

"The doctors at the hospital did lots of tests," Sally said. "That was a long day."

Earl had agreed to be taken to the nearest emergency room, to make sure that he hadn't had a stroke. The CT scan showed no signs of stroke, bleeding, or tumors; however, the doctors suspected that he might have early-stage "small vessel disease," which was common in certain types of dementia. They checked his urine to make sure it wasn't infected and did some basic blood tests, which all came back normal. After a few hours, Earl seemed essentially back to his regular self, so the doctors sent him home with Sally and April with the advice not to drive until he had followed up with his primary care doctor.

"And then it looks like your primary care physician, Dr. Wilson, ordered some additional blood tests," I said, mentioning them by name.

We'd been taught in medical school to perform what our supervisors called a "reversible dementia workup," which included testing for severe thyroid abnormalities, vitamin B_{12} deficiency, and sexually transmitted infections (specifically syphilis).

"Yes, we were told that all of those results were normal too," April said.

I didn't mention the questions that Dr. Wilson had asked Earl to assess his short-term memory, attention span, and other cognitive functions. Those results were abnormal.

I asked April why Dr. Wilson didn't send Earl to a neurologist, since, on the whole, that specialty tended to be more involved with diagnosing dementia than psychiatrists. Or transfer his primary care to a geriatrician, since they, too, were quite familiar with dementia.

"He told us that we could see a neurologist or a psychiatrist," April replied. "That they both deal with diagnosing and treating . . ."

She looked at me, her eyes clouding. She couldn't bring herself to say *Alzheimer's* or *dementia*. At least not in front of her dad. Sally looked away and tugged at the strap on her purse. Earl smiled, seemingly oblivious to the gravity of the moment.

April had called both clinics and was able to get in our clinic sooner. We spent the next few minutes talking about Earl's recent health issues. She described what sounded like progressive mental decline over several months: forgetting familiar names more often, burning a dinner or two, uncharacteristically missing a credit card payment. She probably would have kept providing more details about Earl, but, unexpectedly, he interrupted us.

"It's not as bad as she makes it sound," he said. "I'm doing pretty good. I still cut the grass, and I like working in my garden. I'm old, but I'm not dead yet."

Without realizing it, we had quickly shifted to discussing Earl as though he were a small child in a pediatrician's office or a physically incapacitated person in the medical ICU, when it was clear that he was neither.

"I'm sorry that I haven't been talking to you much," I said. "Can I go through some questions we often ask people that are on the older side and have similar situations?"

"Sure thing," he said. "Whatever you think is good, Doc."

I opened a desk drawer and removed a single sheet of paper, a pre-printed cognitive screening test used in many health care settings. It contained a series of questions that patients needed to answer or tasks they had to perform, all testing different aspects of intellectual functioning. One involved drawing a clock with the two arrows to designate a certain time. Another required starting with the number one hundred and doing serial subtractions by seven. The most anxiety-provoking measure, for many people, was repeating five unrelated objects and recalling those same names five minutes later.

Earl had done a slightly different test with his primary care doctor, so I wanted to try this other one, hoping that maybe he'd had a bad day and would perform better for me. My hopes were quickly dashed as he stumbled on one task after another.

"I was never a great student," he said. "And that was a long time ago."

Sally and April looked increasingly uncomfortable as we proceeded. I wanted to stop, but had to complete it to make a real comparison to the initial test he'd done. Still, by the end, it felt cruel, the same way it would for a teacher to single out a student in class and persistently ask questions that the student couldn't answer.

"Okay," I said finally after I had finished up the test and scored the results. "It looks like what we got today is consistent with what Dr. Wilson got."

"So where does that leave us?" April asked, her expression gloomy.

"There are different types of cognitive impairment," I said. "I'm going to take all of this information I have and discuss it with my supervisor and get back to you later today."

I was just as uncomfortable saying *dementia* or *Alzheimer's* aloud as she was. *Cognitive impairment* sounded medical enough to obscure the impact of what I meant.

"Should we have brought him in sooner?" April asked as she fidgeted in her seat. "He had a scheduled appointment with Dr. Wilson soon, and we were going to bring up the changes then. Maybe we should have been more insistent on bringing Dad in sooner."

April had mentioned that Earl had been showing early signs of mental decline for more than three months. She and Sally looked intently at me.

"I don't think it would have changed anything over the long term," I said. "Not at all."

I didn't want to saddle them with any additional grief or guilt. Besides, from what I knew about dementia and its limited treatments, a few months' delay in diagnosis wasn't going to alter the overall trajectory of his illness, certainly not in the way that detecting lung cancer at stage I versus stage III or IV could completely change someone's future prospects.

"Thank you," Sally said. "We look forward to hearing from you soon."

I called Sally back later that day after I spoke with Dr. Davenport, my supervisor. We agreed to hold off on starting any medications until our follow-up visit in two weeks. That would give her time to talk with April and with friends whose families had been affected by similar problems, she told me. And it would allow me the same to look into possible clinical trial options targeting dementia.

Despite my best intentions, though, I became consumed with other clinical duties and didn't think about Earl or his family again until an hour before his second visit, when I reviewed my schedule for that afternoon. Frantic, I called faculty members that I knew in geriatric psychiatry and neurology to see if they were aware of any clinical studies recruiting participants, but none answered on short notice. When Earl, Sally, and April walked in my office minutes later, I dreaded telling them I hadn't looked into what I'd promised them I would. Thankfully, April had done the homework for me.

"We asked around, and we don't think a clinical trial is for us," she said.

"There's a fifty percent chance he won't get any treatment," Sally chimed in. "And we want to be sure that he's getting something that might help him as soon as possible."

She was referring to the placebo-controlled method, where one group receives the active study treatment (e.g., medications, diet, exercise) and the other group does not; the groups are then compared on some data point—how much they improve on a test of brain function, for example—to determine if the treatment is potentially helpful.

With a clinical study ruled out, I asked them if they wanted me to make a referral to a neurologist or geriatric psychiatrist. Despite Dr. Davenport's earlier guidance, I was still trying to find a way to send them elsewhere. I didn't feel competent to handle his problem.

"Would that change anything as far as starting a medicine for him?" April asked.

I tried to come up with a complex-sounding explanation to convince them—and myself—of the need for a subspecialist referral, but my mind went blank. Prescribing one of the handful of drugs used for dementia, at least at the outset, was actually pretty simple.

"No," I said honestly. "Not at this stage."

"We'd prefer to stay with you," Sally said. "It gets hard to keep seeing new doctors."

Sally seemed to like me. I sensed it after our first meeting. For a brief moment, I allowed myself to be heartened as a young black doctor receiving this warmth from an elderly white woman and her middle-aged daughter. But I quickly switched back to "doctor mode."

"Okay," I said, looking at Earl. "What do you think about taking a medication that could possibly help with . . . maybe remembering things a little better?"

"I feel good," he said. "But I'm fine with it. I already take a pill for blood pressure and another for cholesterol. One more ain't gonna kill me."

Sally mentioned a drug she'd come across in a newspaper article that reportedly had done wonders for an older woman in the early stages of memory loss. What I'd learned in residency suggested otherwise, that these medications had modest benefits at best, and stories such as what Sally mentioned were genuine outliers.

"Okay, that sounds like a good plan," I said.

"We've also been reading about the Mediterranean diet," April said. "There's been some reports that it can help too."

I'd heard a news story or two about the Mediterranean diet, something about how it might reduce the risk for heart disease and increase overall life span. But education on the impact of nutrition on health had been sparse throughout medical school and even less so in my psychiatry training. Unless obesity, diabetes, or hypertension were specific concerns, I rarely, if ever, talked to patients about their diets. That never seemed totally right to me, but the medical model I'd been trained under focused on "evidence-based" approaches, and that "evidence" mostly centered on medications and procedures.

"It certainly can't hurt," I said. "It's definitely worth a try."

I then thought back to my conversation with Dr. Davenport about the important "nonmedical" aspects of dementia. I checked in on my most glaring concern.

"Any updates as far as driving goes?" I asked.

One of my first patients as a psychiatry resident on our university hospital service was an eightysomething woman with dementia who drove for several miles on the wrong side of a local interstate highway. Thankfully, traffic was light that particular day, and police were able to pull her over before anyone was injured. Earl had come to medical attention for confused driving too, so I feared not only for his safety and other motorists, but my own legal liability if he kept on behind the wheel after I'd diagnosed him with dementia.

Earl, April, and Sally all exchanged a few glances before Sally turned back to me.

"We've found a good solution," she said, explaining that Earl agreed to stop driving.

I felt a wave of relief course through my neck and shoulders. "What changed?"

"Drivin' with her isn't peaceful," Earl said, pointing at Sally. "When you get to my age, you need some peace."

We all laughed. Sally said she didn't like driving much herself, so they'd arranged for one of Earl's nephews—one who'd recently retired—to transport Earl around.

"They yap about sports the whole time," Sally said.

"He played football for NC State," Earl said excitedly.

So far, I'd either "talked around" Earl or "talked down" to him, like he was incapacitated or a toddler. Earl's enthusiasm prompted me to try something different.

"Are you a big football fan?" I asked.

He smiled. "I follow whatever's in season. Football. Basketball. Baseball. Golf too."

Sally said he read the daily sports section but never looked at any other part of the newspaper. That sounded exactly like my dad.

"You have a favorite team?" I asked him.

Earl smiled again, bigger this time. He started talking. And talking. But not in a rambling, confused, or disjointed way that I'd seen with patients who had severe dementia or were in the midst of psychosis or mania. Instead, during our ensuing back-and-forth, he tapped into an earlier part of his life, one that admired the athletic feats of 1950s- and 1960s-era stars like Jim Brown, Wilt Chamberlain, and Mickey Mantle to more recent icons like Joe Montana, Larry Bird, and Derek Jeter. Sally and April seemed content, maybe even happy, listening to our exchange, as it reminded them that an important part of their husband and dad was still largely there, even though things had changed considerably and would continue to do so into the future. Before I knew it, nearly ten minutes had passed, and it was almost time for my next appointment. We hadn't done a single "medical" thing during this exchange, but it felt like progress still.

Finally, I shifted focus to discuss medication options. We reviewed his medical history again, and I told them about the more common side effects from this class of dementia drugs. I said that it might improve his mental functioning in the short term or delay his likely cognitive decline, allowing him to remain independent longer. Or it might not do anything at all. In that case, I mentioned a second option we could try. From the prescription standpoint, that was all I could do. They seemed satisfied.

"Thank you again," April said as they all stood to leave.

"It was good talking to you," Earl said. "I hope you have a fine day."

April and Earl continued down the hallway as Sally spun around and approached me.

"He really likes you," she said. "Thanks for talking with him like that and spending time answering all our questions."

As she left, I thought again about my interaction with them: a young black doctor advising an old white couple who'd been my age—early thirties—during the era of segregation. Maybe they had been on the side of the civil rights activists, or, more likely, part of the "moderate" middle. Or maybe, just maybe, they had been on that other side I didn't want to think about. What mattered to me in that moment, though, was the trust that they showed in my role as their doctor, when they certainly had other options.

Race relations aside, my second meeting with Earl allowed me to see him more as an individual and less as a disease process in a medical textbook. Maybe it wouldn't be so bad to have him as a regular patient for as long as that made sense. In fact, I looked forward to his next appointment. We had more sports to discuss.

I TREATED EARL SEVERAL YEARS AFTER MY MEDICAL SCHOOL TEAM took care of Mr. Wilcox, the elderly man with dementia and pneumonia I had been encouraged to avoid. During those in-between years of my medical education, treating patients had been disease-focused, crisis-focused, and hospital-focused. While every competent doctor must learn to work in this way, my encounters with Earl showed how much had been missing in my earlier instruction.

By the time Mr. Wilcox was admitted to our medical service to treat his pneumonia, his cognitive problems had been worsening for years. The man my resident supervisors met was a profoundly diminished version of his former self. He triggered our greatest fears about loss of independence and identity, which no doubt influenced their admonitions that I steer clear of him because he was "not a good teaching case." Had those doctors-in-training encountered him at an earlier point in his mental decline, they might have better appreciated the person beyond the disease. But our medical education hadn't been designed to highlight these aspects of people or to foster those sorts of doctor-patient connections.

The acute care model we trained under worked great for certain sorts of problems—heart attacks, broken bones, appendicitis—that were amenable to drugs or surgeries. However, it delivered less stellar results for patients with chronic diseases, especially those in socially marginalized populations, such as the homeless, the mentally ill, and people with drug addiction. If anything, crisis-oriented medical settings reinforced and perpetuated stereotypes about these and other "second-class" groups, as we repeatedly saw such individuals in their worst moments, rather than on a spectrum of a fuller life.

The same was true with elderly patients. To explore this subject further, I spoke with San Francisco geriatric specialist Dr. Louise Aronson, author of the highly acclaimed *Elderhood*, a 2019 book that confronts, head-on, our long-standing and pervasive biases toward old people, both within medicine and larger society.

"The hospital settings where we train bring us up close to older people who are more frail and prone to bad outcomes," she told me. "This conditions us to think of old people in more negative terms, even when our medical school professors—or someone in our own family—is just as old as that patient, and is doing well."

Indeed, some of the medical professors I admired most were over seventy, and I rejoiced in sharing their company over lunch or in their offices as they told stories about how medicine, and race relations, had evolved during their lives. In my personal life, I had a great-aunt rapidly approaching eighty, who had been a mother figure to my mom after my grandmother's death. She had long-standing orthopedic problems that hindered her gait, and had started showing early signs of cognitive impairment, but, to me, she was simply "Aunt Bee," someone whose company I enjoyed and who loved seeing me. However, in the hospital settings when I encountered an ailing older person, I didn't think of these professors or Aunt Bee. Instead, I saw a man or woman who reflected in my mind how old people were more confused, more difficult to treat, and likelier to die sooner.

My clinical year of medical school did provide one opportunity to meet elderly patients outside the hospital: a one-month rotation at a family medicine clinic. But the four-week stint meant that I saw each patient just once, with no chance to follow their care. Seeing a half dozen elderly patients in relatively good health for fifteen-minute visits did little to counter the experience of seeing a barrage of sick ones hospitalized for weeks during the six-plus months I spent on medicine, surgery, and neurology units. From that skewed vantage point, the old people I saw on my family medicine rotation felt like aberrations, when in fact they were closer to the norm across everyday life.

"We needed a better balance between hospital medicine and outpatient medicine," Dr. Aronson told me, referring to the structure of medical education. "Most patients, most of the time, are not in the hospital."

I didn't know this during the years that I trained in the late 1990s and early 2000s, but a movement was afoot to reform the way that doctors had been educated for nearly a century, both in America and abroad. Dubbed the Longitudinal Integrated Clerkship, or LIC for short, this approach enables students to follow individual patients over time as they receive medical treatment. For example, instead of meeting a pregnant woman at the time of her delivery and having no contact with her afterward, a medical student would get to know some women patients earlier in their pregnancies, attend their labor and delivery, and follow up with them in clinic after they left the hospital. The focus of the program extended beyond learning about a disease or medical treatment to establishing a therapeutic connection over time with patients.

Most of the early LIC programs were geared toward rural settings and outpatient family medicine doctors, but as the model has shown practical benefits to students without compromising their performance on traditional metrics of academic progress, the LIC approach has spread to urban locales and incorporated medical specialists within major hospitals. Between 2010 and 2016, the number of US medical schools offering LIC programs increased by 60 percent; more have been established in the years since, with no signs of this movement receding, despite the added logistical challenges it presents.

By the time I met Earl during the second half of my psychiatry training, I'd finished most of the acute care requirements and was preparing for the remaining year-plus, which largely followed this LIC model. But that transition had arrived dangerously late: my formative experiences in medical school, medical internship year, and the first half of psychiatry residency had conditioned me to think of patients much more as medical illnesses to be solved, rather than as people whose health problems needed our attention. This certainly would have come as sobering news to Sir William Osler, among the most revered and influential physicians of the late nineteenth and early twentieth centuries, who'd famously stated, "The good physician treats the disease; the great physician treats the patient who has the disease." Many of us in medicine had decided that being "good" was just fine.

Dr. Aronson feels that this tunnel-vision approach to medical care particularly fails older people. "Medical school gives us years of training in adult care, months in pediatrics, and just hours or days in the care of old people," she told me. "The result is that doctors feel less competent at helping older patients and help them less effectively, blaming old age for our failures of training and competence. The bad outcomes make us more pessimistic about caring for older patients, and often doctors want to avoid them altogether. It's a self-defeating and self-perpetuating cycle."

Ultimately, Dr. Davenport, my supervisor the day that I met Earl and his family, helped begin to shift my perspective at a crucial professional juncture. He instructed me not to pass off Earl's case to a neurology or geriatric psychiatry clinic, as I desperately wanted. Did he simply think that a general psychiatrist needed good training in evaluating and treating dementia? Or had he seen in me a growing cynicism common among medical trainees that he wanted to confront head-on? Either way, without his actions, I would have missed out on a vital lesson in doctoring.

EARL GOT WORSE OVER TIME, AS WE ALL KNEW WOULD HAPPEN. His mind betrayed him first, and then, ultimately, his body did too. The medication I prescribed—in combination with the dietary changes he'd made—seemed to help some for about three months, or perhaps our collective hope that it would colored our perspective. When his decline became more apparent, around six months after that, I added a second prescription, a newer drug thought to be more effective in the middle and later stages of dementia. It too seemed to help for a few months until it didn't.

Doctors often track cognitive decline through clinic "brain tests" such as the one I'd done with Earl at our first meeting. But I had all the information I needed from observing his increasing detachment from sports. At first, he could no longer watch an entire game, and then not a half, and then not even a quarter (or in the case of baseball, a single inning). Similarly, the daily sports section he'd read his entire adult life steadily became a jumble of pictures, words, and numbers without meaning. Sally, April, and I mourned each step down this cold, thick, uneven terrain, always fearful of when we might step off a cliff.

As my residency graduation approached, we decided on a plan to transition Earl's care to a geriatric psychiatrist. He'd started to develop behavioral symptoms—increasing confusion, irritability, occasional paranoia—that often come with progressive dementia. On the day of his last clinic appointment with me, nearly eighteen months after our first meeting, Earl could still dress and feed himself, but much of what had made him unique had eroded. Yet all was not lost for their family. Sally and April shared how this experience had brought them closer to one another, recapturing the bond they'd shared during April's childhood.

Earl's other daughter, who'd been distant from them for many years, also made overtures to reconnect with her mom and sister.

"Good luck with your career," Sally said with tears in her eyes as she stood to leave my office for the last time. "You're going to make a great doctor."

I thought back to how I'd tried to pass their case off to another doctor, any doctor, immediately after that first visit. I couldn't tell her that, but those feelings compelled me to speak more openly than I did with most patients and families.

"It's been great getting to know you all," I said to each of them, including Earl, who smiled somewhat vacantly back at me. "I've learned so much about life from you all."

Over the next several months, Earl and his family slowly drifted from my thoughts as I adapted to a new job where I saw lots of patients in clinics, the emergency area, and the hospital unit. Life outside work was hectic too; within a year of finishing training, my first child was born.

When I arrived at my office after a largely sleepless night of baby duty, I opened my email inbox to find a note from an administrative clerk I'd worked with during my residency training. April had phoned and asked that I return her call. I assumed there could only be one reason she'd contact me, which April confirmed when I dialed her number during my lunch break.

"I just wanted to let you know that Daddy passed last month," she said. "Mom and I thought you should know given how long you saw him for."

"I'm sorry to hear that," I said, unable to come up with another response.

He was about two and a half years out from that fateful car ride, and I knew that people with dementia often lived much longer, sometimes a decade or more, after diagnosis. I wondered if he had died from suicide, or had an accident.

She told me that Earl had been hospitalized on the psychiatry unit six months earlier after becoming increasingly paranoid and agitated at home following a complicated joint infection. He was then sent to a dementia-care unit, as April and Sally could no longer safely care for him. I thought about the psychiatry residents and medical students who might have seen him in the hospital and how likely their impression of him differed from my own.

"He came down with pneumonia and later sepsis," April continued. "And his body couldn't handle it."

Those last few months had been difficult. But it could have gone on for much longer, with multiple hospital visits and painful medical interventions. Certainly, though, it wasn't my place to say that to April. Thankfully, what she said next let me know she felt the same.

"Mom and I feel like it was for the best. Now he is at peace."

I paused a few seconds before speaking again. "How is your mom?"

"She was in the hospital herself for a week for an irregular heartbeat."

I felt my chest clench ever so slightly. Only near the end of my training did I began to appreciate how difficult the task of caregiving was for spouses and other family, and how this added stress could worsen their health too.

"But she's doing much better now," April said. "They expect her to fully recover."

April told me that her mom was going to sell the house she'd shared with Earl for decades and move in with April and her husband. She then asked how I was doing. I told her that I was a new father.

"Congratulations," she said. "I'm so happy for you."

I looked at my watch. My next patient was in the waiting room. I told April to give my best to Sally. With that send-off, our conversation ended, trading news about one life ending and another beginning. It seemed a fitting symmetry for our relationship as doctor, patient, and caretaking family.

Later that week, I called my mom. It had been a dozen years since my grandmother's death and almost as long since we'd talked about her final days. But April's call made it seem the perfect time. Within minutes, my mom was recounting some details that sounded familiar, but others I felt that I was hearing for the first time. I'd always thought the major stroke had caused my grandmother's dementia, but my mom told me she'd been showing signs of mental decline at least a year earlier than that. She'd even taken it upon herself to start paying her mom's bills.

"Why didn't you tell me?" I asked.

I recalled Earl in his early stages of cognitive impairment and April's initial fear that she'd waited too long to bring him to the doctor.

"I'm sure I did," my mom said, "but you were in your own world back then."

She was right. I was in college an hour away, and my overriding focus was on getting As in my classes and preparing for the MCAT; outside of this premed existence, basketball consumed the rest of my life.

"That's true," I acknowledged.

Now, on the other side of medical training, still career-driven, and with a newborn added in, how much had things really changed for me?

"Have you and Dad talked about getting older?" I began, my voice hesitant. "And how you'd want everything to go if things were to change for either of you, health-wise?"

My mom was then in her late sixties and my dad had just turned seventy. They'd both been in good health to that point, but came from families with many premature deaths.

"Of course," she said. "You know how I like to plan things out."

Indeed, after listening to her explain the finer points of long-term care insurance, Medicare, retirement accounts, and delegation of health care decision-making, it was apparent that she'd thought a lot about what the future might hold, as much as one could given the inherent uncertainty of life. This call marked the first time I'd had a real conversation with my mom about what it could mean for her or my dad to become sick, and how that might impact my older brother and me. I told her how important she and my dad had been to me over the years.

"Sounds like you've finally done some growing up," she said in her loving yet sarcastic style. "I guess you did listen to us at some point."

Becoming a doctor hadn't made me better at dealing with sickness and death; if anything, the lessons from medical school, internship year, and early psychiatry training framed them as things to fear, to avoid whenever possible. In that regard, my experiences with Earl, Sally, and April had been nothing short of transformative. Instead of seeing my future patients with dementia and other debilitating illnesses merely as problems

I'd just as soon avoid, I made greater efforts to see them like Earl, in the early stages of his decline, when we shared our mutual passion for sports. Whenever possible, I tried to engage their families, to help them cope with what they had already lost and would continue to lose, and to guide them toward what they might gain from the arduous journey. Until there is a cure for this dehumanizing disease and others like it, each step that doctors and other medical personnel can make to humanize our patients offers a powerful measure of hope for us all.

8

DIAGNOSE AND TREAT

ERICA FELT WORSE AFTER LEAVING THE DOCTOR'S OFFICE. MUCH worse. A part of her had always feared doctors and the bad news they brought. Diabetes. Dialysis. Dementia. Those had been the words physicians used to label her father, describing his transformation from church deacon and soccer coach in her childhood to a sickly man dead at sixty-eight. The physician she'd just seen had also given her a dreaded "d-word" label: depression. Only now, he'd qualified that initial verdict, telling her that her depression was part of something bigger. Something scarier.

"I thought I was going to lose everything," she later told me. "Everything."

Her first appointment with him had taken place a month earlier. Like many people—probably most—she never imagined winding up in a psychiatrist's office, crying to a stranger. But life had "snuck up" on her. As she approached forty, she'd had a failed marriage, two miscarriages, and a career as a high school teacher that seemed stuck in neutral. Her dad died the year before, and for reasons she didn't fully understand, she'd become estranged from her younger sister. After she made an embarrassing scene at her mother's birthday party, she called in sick to her boss and stayed in bed for three days. Her mom told her she needed professional help.

A coworker helped her schedule with a psychiatrist who accepted her health insurance. The appointment lasted thirty minutes. She cried a lot. He told her she had both depression and anxiety disorders, and prescribed her three different medications. One was for depression. One was for anxiety. One was for sleep. The way that he explained this made sense to her in his office, but she began having doubts on the drive home. *Three* medicines? Was she so bad off, she wondered, that one pill, or even two, couldn't do?

I first heard about Erica's plight from Dr. Wang, a primary care doctor, who stood at the entryway to the office that I used on Tuesdays. I turned my rolling chair toward her.

"I have someone new I need help with," she told me. "Can you see her?"

I had finished my psychiatry residency the previous year and now worked two days a week at a VA medical clinic located forty minutes from the VA hospital where I'd trained. Primary care services were offered on one side of the building and mental health treatment on the other. Although many people on the primary care wing had mental health needs, and nearly all the ones on our side had general medical concerns, a patient very rarely saw both of us on the same day. The only exceptions occurred if we had someone with active chest pain or another acute medical crisis. And the primary care doctors only requested same-day service from us for someone suicidal, psychotic, or manic whom they felt was unsafe to leave the clinic without immediate psychiatric input. Months went by without patients crossing this invisible line.

"What's going on with her?" I asked Dr. Wang.

"I'm not sure if she's suicidal," Dr. Wang replied, "but she's a mess right now. She's on a bunch of psych drugs, and I have no idea what's going on. I can't send her out like this."

"She come alone?" I asked. "Or is someone with her who could take her to the ER?"

I was trained to think through worst-case scenarios. Ambulance services sometimes refused to transport people from clinics who had psychiatric emergencies, citing concerns about protocols and safety. Psychiatric patients were too much trouble, it seemed. Often, we relied on a patient's family member or friend to fill that void.

"She's by herself," Dr. Wang said. "She definitely doesn't want to go
to the hospital."

"Has she been to one before? A psych hospital or psych ER?"

Dr. Wang shook her head. "She told me she'd never had any mental
health treatment until a few months ago."

"Who's prescribing her meds?" I asked.

"A private psychiatrist she's seen a few times," she answered as she
glanced at the overhead wall clock. "But it doesn't seem to be helping.
She doesn't want to go back to him."

"You have her med list?"

Dr. Wang handed me a sheet of paper on which she'd written notes.
At her first visit to the psychiatrist, Erica had been prescribed three new
medications. At the second visit a month later, all three were stopped
and she was given four different ones.

"That sounds like a lot of pills even for you guys," Dr. Wang said as
she smiled at me.

I'd known Dr. Wang for almost a year, and we'd had a few lengthy
conversations on hefty topics like immigration, race, and history. I knew
that she respected me, even if she didn't like psychiatry much. So I felt
comfortable counterpunching.

"You guys prescribe too many drugs too," I said, smiling back at her.
"And it's not always based on objective lab tests either."

I always reviewed the current electronic medication record for each
patient I saw, since a handful of prescriptions can worsen (or even cause)
mental health issues, and some psychiatric drugs can have problematic
interactions with other medications. In glancing at these lists, it seemed
that every other patient took pills for chronic back pain or headaches,
and even more for gastric reflux. These conditions relied heavily on patient self-report and often had effective non-medication strategies that
lost out to the ease of prescribing and taking a drug.

"But we're treating the whole body and the whole person," she fired
back. "And unfortunately, they don't give us enough time to do that well.
Nowhere near enough."

Most primary care doctors I knew shared similar sentiments, that they were expected to accomplish too much with too little time and that pre-scribing medications was often necessary to keep the patient flow moving.

"Do you have time to work her in?" she said, as she eyed the wall clock behind me again. "I think she'd be fine in the waiting room. One of the clerks can keep an eye on her."

My clinic days were usually full, but I had an unexpected gap in the schedule. One patient had no-showed and another had canceled, leav-ing me with forty-five minutes before the next appointment. I had some administrative tasks I'd planned to complete in the interim, but those could wait.

"I'll see her now. Do you need this paper?" I asked, referring to her notes.

She shook her head and smiled again. "All yours. My nurse has her vitals. I know she's in good hands. Thanks, Damon."

As Dr. Wang walked away, I began to map out how I envisioned the appointment going. My main goal was to see Erica and evaluate her risk for suicide, or anything else that might warrant an emergency room trip. But I was already brainstorming triage options for her outpatient care going forward. And here, my biases quickly set in. First off, the last few brand-new women veteran patients I'd met had histories of sexual assault and felt uncomfortable with me as their doctor, so I was already think-ing of which woman psychiatrist I could have her see.

But gender was just part of my hesitancy in seeing her. Someone who'd been prescribed seven medications in two visits had to be "complicated," as we described such patients in medicine, and I already had plenty of people on my list who fit that description. These were the patients con-stantly seeking medication changes. The ones who doubled or tripled the prescribed doses on their own. The men and women who invari-ably, it seemed, requested controlled meds and, with that, brought more complexity to their treatments. But in blaming Erica for her medication list, which I was doing without acknowledging it, I was overlooking the obvious: the role of psychiatry and medicine in this larger problem.

———

PSYCHIATRIC DRUGS ARE ENTRENCHED WITHIN MEDICAL PRACTICE
and American society. Over the past decade, between 15 and 20 percent of US residents each year have taken prescription medication for
mental health conditions. Antidepressants (such as sertraline and fluoxetine) and anxiolytics (such as diazepam and alprazolam) rank among
the most widely dispensed categories of drugs, trailing only common
staples such as pain meds, cholesterol-lowering agents, and high blood
pressure pills. Individually, six psychiatric meds made the top-twenty-
five list for the most prescribed drugs of 2020. And while psychiatrists,
such as the one Erica saw, undoubtedly authorize millions of prescriptions annually, the reality is that throughout much of the US, people
are actually more likely to receive these drugs from family doctors, pediatricians, nurse practitioners, gynecologists, and a mishmash of other
medical specialists. The horse is out of the pharmaceutical barn.

I witnessed this explosion as a medical student in the mid-to-late
1990s. Prozac, Zoloft, and Paxil—the early brand-name selective serotonin reuptake inhibitors (SSRIs)—were all in their first decade of existence, and it seemed as if every third patient we admitted to the hospital
with heart disease, cancer, or other malady took one of these medications. Many also took sedatives or sleeping pills.

Working on medical and surgical wards, where the focus was on
more urgent and, to our thinking, more important concerns, the doctors I worked with usually took little interest in this, simply continuing these psych meds for patients in the hospital and leaving it to their
outpatient providers to resume them after discharge. One day, however,
during my round with a general surgery team, psychiatric meds briefly
took center focus.

"Half the women we see these days are on one of these newer depression meds," the senior surgeon said to the male surgery resident, whom
he supervised.

We'd just finished seeing a sixtysomething woman a few days out
from gallbladder surgery. The patient before her was a woman half her
age who'd just had her appendix removed. Both were on antidepressants
started by their family physicians.

"*Prozac Nation*," the junior surgeon replied, referring to a bestselling book published a few years earlier.

"It wasn't like this eight or ten years ago," the senior surgeon said. "The folks on psych meds then were crazies or neurotics. Not nice, regular-looking ladies like this."

Beneath his demeaning language, the surgeon had his finger on a surging trend. Between 1988, the year after Prozac was introduced, and two decades later in 2008, the rate of antidepressant use in the US increased by 400 percent. And women took them more than twice as much as men.

My next rotation at a family medicine clinic gave me an even closer view of the proliferation of psychiatric drugs. One afternoon, I followed my supervisor for the day, Dr. Springer, into the room of a fortysomething woman who reported headaches, fatigue, and insomnia. My eager medical student brain ran through a host of potential endocrine, neurological, and rheumatologic causes for her symptoms. But Dr. Springer spent most of the next ten minutes asking her questions about her job and her family life. She conceded that she felt worn down and had trouble enjoying things like she had in the past. After a cursory physical exam, he rendered his diagnosis.

"Sounds like you're depressed," he said confidently.

The woman glanced at him, her freckled face registering confusion, before she looked down at her folded hands. She seemed uncertain that this was her problem.

Dr. Springer said that depression was a medical condition no different from high blood pressure or high cholesterol. But those illnesses had measurable numbers, I told myself, whereas depression seemed to be based on a checklist of somewhat vague symptoms. To my thinking at the time, hypertension seemed "scientific," whereas depression did not.

"I'm going to give you some samples to try for a month," he continued. "I'll see you then, and we can decide on next steps."

"Okay," the woman said hesitantly. "Thank you, Doctor."

I'd moved on to another rotation by the time of her follow-up visit, but before I left, I saw more than a dozen patients who'd been started on antidepressants within the previous few months. Many said they felt

better. The rest said the medication either didn't help or caused some un-
pleasant side effect. That data more or less mirrored patient responses to
diabetes, high blood pressure, and cholesterol medicines, but I couldn't
fully get past the idea that those conditions had numbers we could measure with laboratory tests, whereas with depression, it seemed we had to
rely almost exclusively on what a patient told us. Could Dr. Springer really be right that identifying and treating depression wasn't so different
from many other medical conditions he saw? It seemed like a stretch.

Still, I carried this perception of psychiatry, that it was most useful
when it prescribed medicines the same way we treated high blood pressure or reflux, throughout medical school, intern year, and ultimately,
into most of my psychiatry residency. On psychiatric units, meds ruled
the day, only the patients took more potent ones like lithium, antipsychotic drugs (e.g., risperidone, quetiapine), and anti-seizure pills (e.g.,
valproic acid, carbamazepine) known as *mood stabilizers*. Many took
several meds in combination. Unlike those patients in the family medicine clinic, however, people often did not fare as well on the medications, and these drugs came with more side effects. But we blamed the
illnesses themselves rather than the treatments, in a similar way I'd seen
oncologists accept the toxicity of chemotherapy agents in the name of
fighting aggressive cancers.

It was only later in my psychiatry training that I began to have doubts
about the prescription-focused approach. While I staffed the mental
health urgent care clinic on a busy Thursday afternoon, a man in his late
thirties came in requesting a "happy pill" like he'd seen on a television
commercial. Because the other resident and I were tied up with patients
who needed hospitalization, our faculty supervisor, Dr. Northson, saw
this man himself. Toward the end of a shift, when things had slowed
down, he told us about this encounter:

"Sometimes I think we're going too far in the other direction," he began. "Medications are essential for very depressed people, but this guy is
just unhappy with his marriage. He needs counseling to make it better
or to decide whether he wants a divorce. Not Zoloft. But those smiling
faces on TV are telling him there's a pill to solve his problems."

Direct-to-consumer advertising of pharmaceutical drugs took off in the late 1990s while I was in medical school, and, by the time I was a psychiatry resident a few years later, it had become a multibillion-dollar effort from leading drug companies.

"Isn't that true for other medical issues too?" asked a psychiatric nurse who worked with us. "That maybe we should try to change our lifestyles first before jumping to pills?"

She raised a good point. Indeed, there were drug ads for all of life's ills, it seemed—erectile problems, hair loss, headaches, joint pains, and many others—with a pervasive message of better living through pharmacotherapy. Dr. Northson countered that mental illnesses were inherently more subjective and thus easier to blur the boundaries of normal and abnormal. A critic might say he was admitting that psychiatric practice was inferior to the "objective" space that the rest of medicine inhabited. But I wondered if what he was telling us instead was that psychiatry's quest to be like the rest of medicine was causing it to lose what made it special.

These thoughts circulated in my mind a few months later as I met Larry, a new patient assigned to my outpatient clinic. He was midtwenties, good-looking, with an athletic build, but he struggled with dating and found himself frustratingly alone most weekends. He didn't like his engineering job much and was thinking of changing careers. When I asked specific questions about depression and anxiety symptoms, he acknowledged problems with both, clearly sounding distressed.

"My friend told me I should try something to take the edge off," he said.

He mentioned a drug called Xanax, which belongs to a class of sedatives called benzodiazepines. Before Xanax became a mainstay in many people's medicine cabinets, Valium, a similar drug, had fulfilled that role for an earlier generation. While these medications definitely eased anxiety, I'd seen too many people in my hospital rotations experience addiction-like problems with their regular use to recommend them as first-line treatments in most cases. Especially for someone like Larry, whose dad and uncle were both excessive alcohol drinkers. I explained my concerns.

"Yeah, I guess I don't need that," Larry said, shaking his head. He then offered his second choice. "My friend also mentioned a drug called Lexapro. What do you think about that?"

Lexapro was a newer option in the Prozac, Paxil, and Zoloft orbit, marketed as having fewer side effects than its predecessors.

"Sure," I said without much conviction.

"That's what I'd like to try then," he said.

From what I was learning in my weekly psychotherapy seminar, our instructors—mostly psychologists—would have suggested Larry consider talk therapy first. With that approach, he might get a deeper understanding of his dating anxieties or develop a concrete plan to chart his next career steps. But I had a lot more experience prescribing medications, and that was what Larry pushed for in any case: a pill to calm him and improve his outlook without digging into the details of his inner life. Prescribing a drug seemed the easier path, for both doctor and patient. Lexapro to the rescue. I would see him back in a month.

As I sat down to enter a medical note in his electronic record, I thought about the periods in my life when I felt uncertainty and discontent: college, when my basketball exploits hadn't panned out as I'd hoped; med school, when I questioned whether I'd made the right career choice; intern year, when I decided to forgo my goal to become a cardiologist, and later found myself in the office of a clinical social worker. Should I have been on medications at each phase to ease my distress? Or had I emerged from those setbacks with renewed focus and motivation? Would life have turned out differently, for better or for worse, with meds? Of course, there was no way to run things back and conduct that test. What struck me most as I typed Larry's note was that the idea to take medication never crossed my mind. What did that say about me and my thoughts about mental health? About Larry and others like him?

Completing Larry's medical note required me to enter "diagnosis and procedure codes," a necessity so the clinic could bill his health insurance company and get paid. The procedure part was straightforward; he was a new patient I'd seen for a set amount of time for a psychiatric assessment, so I checked off the box that best fit those descriptors. The diagnosis portion was trickier. Psychiatric diagnoses were based on something called the *Diagnostic and Statistical Manual of Mental Disorders* (*DSM*), then in its fourth edition (text revision), which spelled out checklist criteria for hundreds of psychiatric disorders. Larry didn't really fit neatly into any category; something called an Adjustment Disorder seemed best. But prescribing a daily medication seemed to require a robuster diagnosis than that, so I went with the slightly less vague Anxiety Disorder, Not Otherwise Specified. And just like that, I'd given Larry a label and a pill for it, the same way many physicians then identified low back pain or headache and prescribed pain meds. Or gave acid blockers for reflux. Diagnose and treat (with drugs) was what we as doctors had been taught to do.

I pushed aside any reservations I had about this treatment approach when I chose my first job after finishing residency training. Outpatient clinics suited me better temperamentally than working on an inpatient unit where the patients were sicker. And so I settled into a medical office where new patients came to me in one of two ways: from a primary care doctor's referral, or at the recommendation of a mental health therapist (social worker or psychologist) who saw the person first. In either scenario, the purpose in meeting me was to evaluate whether someone would benefit from "medication management" of their mental health symptoms. My role in the mental health ecosystem was to prescribe drugs.

"It's a practice that's very reminiscent of primary care," said Dr. Steven S. Sharfstein, a former president of the American Psychiatric Association, in a 2011 *New York Times* article exploring psychiatry's shift from psychotherapy to medication management, published a few years after I'd started working at the clinic. "They check up on people," he continued, "they pull out the prescription pad; they order tests."

Despite the hand-wringing nature of the article, this model initially suited me fine. After all, I'd gone to medical school and spent a year as a medical intern with the goal of becoming a cardiologist, a specialty, like most in medicine, where monitoring vital signs, performing physical exams, ordering labs and other tests, and prescribing meds were the foundation of care. Why should psychiatry, given that so many general medical conditions were known to cause mental distress, be different?

Especially if medication seemed to help many patients and was their preferred treatment of choice.

A year into this job, however, those doubts from my residency training resurfaced. One morning, I saw a man in his fifties transferred to me from another doctor who'd recently moved to another state. His chart listed post-traumatic stress disorder (PTSD), a common diagnosis in this clinic. But his medication list wasn't ordinary, at least not to my thinking.

"Are you taking each one?" I asked him, assuming that some of the six listed were previous medications that hadn't been deleted from his record.

The man said he took four of them (two antidepressants and two mood stabilizers) daily, the fifth (an antianxiety pill) just about every day, and the sixth (a sleeping pill) at least three times each week.

"Do they seem to be helping?"

His answer amounted to "somewhat." He felt less anxious overall and slept better, but he mostly kept to himself. I asked whether he had tried psychotherapy, which can be especially effective in treating PTSD.

"They tried to put me in a group once," he replied. "I didn't take to that."

We talked about other psychotherapy options, but he didn't seem eager for change. Soon, time ran low, and I needed to figure out what to do with his meds. He told me he'd consider various adjustments in the future but that, for now, he wanted to keep it the same. He'd been on this regimen for over a year and felt better than when he started. So we left it as is. Still, as I renewed these prescriptions, I worried about various drug interactions that I discussed with him, including unintentional overdose, and long-term side effects such as weight gain, heart-related concerns, and internal bleeding. But maybe if someone was willing to assume all these risks taking medications, I told myself, this meant the other side—life without them—was substantially worse. Who was I to judge him for that?

I soon saw that this psychiatric polypharmacy approach wasn't so unusual. About two years after starting my full-time day job, with one infant son and another on the way, I picked up some weekend shifts at a private psychiatric hospital. There, one morning, a short, soft-spoken man in his early sixties arrived for what his chart described as "uncontrollable anxiety." When I met him in an admitting-area exam room, he handed me a standard-size sheet of white paper.

"This is what I'm taking," he said.

I looked down and thought my eyes were going to pop out of their sockets. The list was a Noah's ark of psychiatric medications: two antidepressants, two mood stabilizers, two antipsychotic drugs, two antianxiety medications, and two sleeping pills.

"All of them?" I asked, disbelieving.

He nodded. How could a doctor prescribe that many meds in duplicate? My first thought was that this patient should have been hospitalized sooner. Maybe he needed ECT? Or intensive psychotherapy? Or at least a second opinion? But since he wasn't suicidal, the patient told me that his previous health insurer wouldn't cover hospitalization. And none of the therapists recommended to him accepted his insurance. So prior to him getting new health coverage, both patient and doctor had gone down the path of adding more and more drugs, an approach that his health insurance, operating under the "psychiatrist as pill-prescriber model," did cover. I tried to imagine myself in a clinical situation where prescribing nearly a dozen meds seemed my only recourse to address a patient's emotional distress. I'd probably quit if it came to that.

Tempted as some might be to pin all this irresponsible prescribing on psychiatrists, I admitted other patients on later weekends who came in on equally worrisome drug regimens—mixes of stimulants, benzodiazepines, and antipsychotics—started by primary care doctors and neurologists. Even a dermatologist and a cardiologist joined the gathering. One woman got her back surgeon into the fold. It seemed that no specialty was immune.

By the time I saw Erica that morning, I'd grown increasingly disillusioned about my work as a psychiatrist. Many patients, likely influenced by pharmaceutical advertising and our collective desire for quick fixes, only wanted medication treatments. And that had become all I felt comfortable providing them in any case, as the psychotherapy skills I developed in residency receded. Erica, with seven prescribed pills over two visits, appeared next up on this assembly line. But what at first looked like another case of "medication management" helped me reimagine how I could help people as a psychiatrist.

"YOU'RE REALLY TALL," ERICA SAID TO ME, HER VOICE TIMID, AS we entered my office area. "Your head is close to that doorway. I'm not used to feeling short very often."

Erica had on flat shoes and looked about five ten or five eleven. Virtually every day that I met new people, at least one person commented on my height. I assumed correctly that she'd ask me about basketball next, but she brought up the topic with a twist.

"I have a student who is about your size," she continued, sounding more assured. "Everyone around my school is saying he should focus on basketball to get into college, but I think it could do wonders for him to see someone like yourself who is a doctor."

The connection between height and basketball success is obvious, but I sensed the subtext here involved race. I was black, Erica was black, and I assumed her student was too. Given the acclaim some black men have achieved in the game, people often assume that it is the best path for any black kid with any sort of athletic inclination. Yet only a tiny fraction are able to carve out a living on the hardwood.

"What do you teach?"

"American history. That can be dicey for us," she said, once again, I presumed, making a racial reference. "I think I do the best I can."

Many visits I had with patients began with small talk. I told myself that it was for their benefit, to help them ease into discussing their worries and despair. But I needed it also, to remind me that the people I saw weren't just problems to patch up and send along, as I increasingly felt in my current work; rather, they were real individuals with lives outside the walls of a psychiatric office. Without knowing it, Erica had briefly touched on four things I cared about deeply—race, basketball, education, and history. I found myself feeling a bit calmer as I switched into doctor mode.

"Dr. Wang told me a little about what brought you here today," I began.

Erica broke eye contact, looking down at her hands. She started rubbing her thumbs, and then she picked off lint from her beige pants. She'd just met me, and now she had to share what she probably liked least about herself.

"I'm not sure what's wrong," she said. "I've sort of lost control of my life."

I glanced at the digital time on the computer monitor. Ideally, I would have asked her what that felt like and when she thought this change started, but I needed to get to the crux of why Dr. Wang had broken our clinic's invisible barrier between primary care and mental health services and asked me to see Erica. My job was triage.

"Have you thought about ending your life," I asked, "or hurting yourself directly in some other way?"

Erica met my eyes briefly before focusing on something behind me. "No, nothing quite that bad. Sometimes I do question why I'm here, though. And maybe that my mom would be better off if . . . if I weren't around. I don't want to actually kill myself, though."

Some people downplayed thoughts about suicide out of shame, or fearing it would bring about a trip to the emergency room or a psychiatric hospital. But I had no basis to doubt her.

She swatted at the tear that sloped down her nose. "I'm sorry," she said.

I wanted to find out more about her family, her job, and all the other stuff that makes up a person's life. However, I needed to focus on the second reason Dr. Wang had brought Erica to me: to sort out her medication list.

After Erica's first visit, the psychiatrist had started her on sertraline (for depression), buspirone (for anxiety) and zolpidem (for sleep). At the second visit, he stopped these three and switched her to lithium and lamotrigine (mood stabilizers), clonazepam (stronger anxiety medicine), and risperidone (an antipsychotic medication). With so many simultaneous additions and changes, how would he or the patient know what worked and what didn't? What caused side effects and what didn't?

"Did the doctor give you a specific diagnosis?" I asked. "Or more than one diagnosis?"

"At the first visit," she replied, "he told me major depression and generalized anxiety. The next time, he said he thought I was bipolar."

With those possibilities in mind, I went through the usual psychiatric interview, one where I asked about her energy levels, sleep patterns, and other symptoms related to one's mood. I inquired whether she had any intense fears or preoccupations, and whether she experienced any unusual perceptions, such as sounds or sights others might not perceive. Did she consume alcohol, marijuana, or other drugs, and if so, how often and how much? Did anyone in her family suffer from mental health or drug-related problems? And so forth.

The process took about ten minutes.

"Did he explain his thinking to you?"

People diagnosed with bipolar disorder have distinct episodes of depression and mania (or hypomania), mental states usually thought to be polar opposites of one another. The condition was initially called *manic-depressive illness*, or simply *manic depression*.

"I couldn't sleep at all after he started me on those first meds. Even though I felt tired, those drugs kept me up. He said that could be a sign that I was bipolar."

I asked more questions about her mood, energy level, and behaviors, both recently and before she started noticing emotional problems. Based on her answers, I felt confident about what she didn't have.

"I think the likelihood that you have what we call bipolar disorder is very low," I told her.

"Are you sure?"

Bipolar disorder, with nonspecific symptoms that can at times be difficult to nail down, can be tricky to diagnose, and as a result, misdiagnosis is common in both directions. Some doctors almost never make the diagnosis, while others assign it liberally. In that regard, the varying approaches seem analogous to the variations in how US Supreme Court justices interpret our Constitution. I tried, as best I could, to stake a middle ground. Based on how I analyzed what she told me, and what the then-current *DSM* listed, Erica's history didn't line up as her having this condition.

"Yes," I said assuredly.

Erica sighed audibly, her shoulders dropping in relief. "Thank you so much. That really scared me. I worried that meant I was eventually going to go crazy and lose my job. My ex-husband's younger brother had that illness, and it ruined his life."

I thought about how bipolar disorder could be perceived differently depending on one's place in the social strata. In elite circles, there was talk about a potential association between mania and creativity, with some authors exploring how the condition likely afflicted famous historical figures in business, politics, and especially the creative arts. However, in the world many poorer people and racial minorities inhabited, being perceived as hyperactive, impulsive, and erratic might get you kicked out of school or locked in prison. Or killed.

Ruling out bipolar disorder didn't mean I knew what label or diagnosis to give her, any more than an emergency medicine doctor does who tells a patient that their chest pain isn't from a heart attack or their dizziness from a stroke. I felt that sorting through the reasons behind Erica's woes required time that I didn't have.

"I'd like to set you up for a follow-up appointment," I said. "With one of our therapists. They can help you talk through how you've been feeling and work on ways to feel better."

Erica's eyes scanned my face as if she were trying to read me. "Okay," she said finally. "What should I do about the medications?"

She had already stopped the risperidone, after reading about its side effects, and was taking only half the prescribed clonazepam dose because of daytime drowsiness. Sometimes we labeled patients like this as being "noncompliant," but she'd chosen wisely. We settled on a much simpler regimen: one antidepressant medicine (bupropion) and one sleeping pill (doxylamine, an antihistamine) that she could purchase over the counter.

"If I saw a therapist, would I still see you?" she asked.

Before meeting Erica, I'd already plotted how to get her scheduled with one of my female psychiatrist colleagues. But for me to do that at this point, after we'd had a perfectly nice interaction, would have been for my convenience, not for her benefit.

"Yes. You'd still need a psychiatrist to prescribe medications," I said, knowing that Dr. Wang, her primary physician, would be disinclined to do so herself.

"So is that how they have it set up here too, where I'd see two different people? That's how it was at the other place. That psychiatrist was going to send me to a therapist once he felt that I was more stable."

"For the most part, we do the same thing here," I replied.

Erica was describing split care, where patients receive combined treatment; they see psychiatrists (or increasingly, mental health nurse practitioners) for prescriptions and nonphysician providers (e.g., psychologists, clinical social workers, and marriage and family therapists) for talk therapy. Over time, this has become the predominant model of mental health care, both in private and public settings, because it is seen as cheaper (nonmedical therapists earn less than psychiatrists), and more efficient in its use of clinical expertise. Some patients seem perfectly fine with this arrangement, while others take more to one clinician over the other, which can complicate treatment.

"I understand," she said. "I guess it's just hard to have to tell the story over again."

I thought back to how our conversation started. Erica was a history teacher invested in encouraging her students to see beyond their present circumstances and society's constraints to imagine a better life. Removed from the psychiatric labels and medications, she reminded me of teachers and school counselors I'd known at various stages of my life, some of whom had undoubtedly helped me carve my own path, one that far exceeded what a sociologist might have projected for me at birth.

"You know what," I began, "let's forget about that. I'll see you back in two weeks. We'll see how the med changes are going and talk more about how you've been feeling."

My clinic schedule booked out at least two months for return visits. That meant I'd have to squeeze Erica into a slot usually carved for administrative time, when I wrote medical notes and returned patient messages. Those things still would need to get done, so I'd have to do them while eating lunch at my desk. Yet given how much teachers and counselors had once helped me, and that I sensed Erica was trying to do the same for the next generation, I pushed aside any misgivings that I had.

"That works," she said. "We're on spring break in three weeks, so I can come then."

I felt a twinge of guilt as we finalized this appointment. That somehow I was playing favorites inappropriately. What about all of the other patients I saw who needed more than prescriptions? Some were suitably established with nonmedical therapists, but these colleagues were in short supply and often booked out further than I did in terms of taking on new referrals. Other patients simply scoffed at the idea of seeing two specialists for what they saw as the same problem. Invariably, some people fell through the cracks.

But as one psychiatrist in a medical clinic that served thousands of patients, I could only do so much. If I overbooked everyone who might need it, I would have added another hour or two to my days and soon found myself teetering ever closer to full-fledged burnout, which seemed to be afflicting an increasing number of doctors across disciplines. *No, I shouldn't feel guilty*, I told myself. The problem wasn't me. It was the American health care system itself, one that seemingly forced its staff to work overtime to deliver good care.

"It was nice talking to you," Erica said as our appointment started to wind down. "The other psychiatrist I saw, he seemed so rushed. Everything he asked me was from a checklist, and he kept cutting me off to stay on his script."

I'd done all the things she described with other patients, increasingly so as I grew more efficient (and cynical); I suspected that some of my patients had said similar things about me to other people. We'd been taught as doctors to follow a script. There didn't seem any other way to manage the barrage of distressed people who came to us. And I'd followed one with Erica too, only she didn't feel that way, probably due to the relief she'd gotten from my assurances that she wasn't "crazy."

As Erica walked away, I thought about how seeing her in clinic during my administrative break was going to make some days extra busy. But maybe, just maybe, it would be worth it, both for her and for me.

AMONG THE MANY CRITIQUES OF PSYCHIATRY, THE MOST FREQUENTLY expressed are its process of diagnosis and treatment. "What exactly is depression?" one might ask. "And who decides whether it is so?" After all, common experience tells us that people can feel sad and hopeless for any number of reasons—a divorce, the death of a child or spouse, getting fired, failing out of school, their kids leaving home for college, moving to a new area and feeling lonely, suffering a severe physical injury, and having a terminal illness, to name some. Or they can start feeling bad "out of the blue" for no apparent reason. There is no blood test (outside of medical conditions known to cause depression, such as hypothyroidism), brain imaging, brain wave analysis, or genetic data that might reliably identify a depressed person from a nondepressed individual. The same limitations apply for bipolar disorder and schizophrenia, even as their severe characteristics seem to argue more strongly for a biomedical cause. Diagnoses are based on patient self-report and physician observation.

With the biology of mental illness not fully understood, it's not surprising that its biological treatments face the greatest criticism. After all, how can we make drugs, of which we remain uncertain how exactly they alleviate emotional distress, the mainstay of treatment, when we are unsure of whether what they are treating is truly a biological illness? Given our lack of certainty about mental illness and psychiatric medications, we should not be surprised that people's responses to these drugs vary so greatly. Some people will find a prescription of fluoxetine transformative, others will feel slightly better but not really well, another group will notice no mental changes at all (although they may experience physical side effects, such as nausea and sex problems), and, finally, the last group will say they feel demonstrably worse—more anxious, more depressed, or "like a zombie."

It is in this framework that critics assert that psychiatrists are not really like the white-coated and scrub-wearing physicians of other disciplines.

But perhaps the true problem is that psychiatrists are trying to be too much like them when their methods, too, are flawed.

For sure, there are medical illnesses that can be objectively defined by X-rays and lab tests—think a broken leg, a heart attack, or a bloodstream infection. In many cases, their treatments can be correspondingly definitive—surgical fixation, bypass surgery, or intravenous antibiotics. Scientific advances such as these and others throughout the twentieth century brought wondrous lifesaving interventions to people fortunate enough to access them, and those of us in the twenty-first century continue to reap the benefits as these technologies and therapies become further refined. By comparison, psychiatry, with its ambiguous assessments and crude treatments, indeed seems stuck in the premodern era.

Yet these exemplars of medical innovation and ingenuity represent a small fraction of addressing the health needs that bring patients to doctors. Most illnesses, in reality, are better characterized as "chronic diseases"—think hypertension, diabetes, and high cholesterol. They often come on gradually and lack a clear-cut cause in the way that acute illnesses usually do, and they tend to stay with us for months, years, often a lifetime, as they elude definitive medical or surgical cures. These diseases are exceedingly common—affecting more than half of the adult population—and are impacted by lifestyle and environment, causing significant disability and premature death. Sound familiar?

Many of these chronic illnesses do have numbers attached to them—virtually all of us have had a blood pressure cuff squeeze our arms, have had a phlebotomist puncture our skin with a needle, and have peed into a sterile cup. But the lines distinguishing sick from well are fuzzier than we might think. Can we say with confidence, for example, that a blood pressure of 131/86 mmHg taken on two random clinic days represents medical illness whereas someone whose numbers are 129/84 mmHg in those same settings is entirely normal (with 130/85 mmHg being the cutoff)? Or that a cholesterol of 201 is appreciably different from a value of 199 (with 200 the cutoff)? Or that a hemoglobin A1C of 6.5 is absolutely diabetes while a value of 6.4 indicates only prediabetes (with 6.5 the cutoff)? Further complicating matters is that the numbers that define certain chronic diseases have shifted over time and likely will continue to be modified into the future. Laboratory results considered normal in 1993 are, in many instances, abnormal in 2023.

And other conditions lack quantitative rigor altogether. Take headaches, which rank among the most common reasons for medical visits throughout the world. A handful are due to what we term "secondary causes," such as a brain tumor, an aneurysm, head trauma, or an infection. Yet most are classified as either tension headaches, which people often experience as a tightening band around their head and neck areas, or migraines, which disproportionately bring headache sufferers to doctors.

Migraines are especially dramatic. They often present as severe, recurrent, pulsating attacks of pain localized to one side of the head that can last for minutes, hours, or days. Nausea and heightened sensitivity to light or sound are common. Some have what we call an aura—sensory changes, visual alterations, or even speech changes that precede the headache. Yet the cause of this unquestionably medical-sounding condition remains largely unknown, its diagnosis reliant on a patient's self-report. In a 2017 *New Yorker* essay profiling a Boston headache specialist, surgeon and writer Atul Gawande described migraines as "a problem invisible to the naked eye, to blood tests, to biopsies, and to scans and often not even believed by co-workers, family members, or indeed, doctors." If I hadn't known the context, I would have thought he was describing the current state of mental illness.

The treatments themselves aren't always concrete either. During my medical internship year, I spent a half day each week in an outpatient primary care clinic attached to the hospital. Most patients were over fifty, with two or more chronic diseases. But Spencer, an HVAC technician in his late twenties, had only one problem: chronic headaches. By the time I met him, he'd been going to a neurology clinic for over a year. Along with over-the-counter drugs, such as acetaminophen (Tylenol) and ibuprofen, they'd started him on a triptan agent, a class of drugs introduced in the 1990s that revolutionized the treatment of migraines by reducing the severity and duration of acute migraine attacks.

And though the triptan medicine helped Spencer in that way ("Fifty percent better," he'd told me), the headache episodes still happened about twice per week. So his doctor took to prescribing an array of as prophylaxis. Some were the same types that psychiatrists used to treat bipolar disorder or had previously used as first-line medication for depression. He'd also taken two different blood pressure pills. Some had side effects; others simply didn't help.

"They just keep pumping me full of these drugs," he said to me at one visit. "But they don't know what's causing it. Maybe I'm just cursed or something."

Despite its life-altering success for some people, the pharmacology-only approach to headaches, much like what I'd later see with psychiatry, clearly had limitations for others. Spencer's self-doubt mirrored Erica's years later, when she felt her psychiatrist seemed to reduce her to labels and pills. But as a doctor in training with limited knowledge and even less time, all I knew to offer Spencer was assurance that I'd let his neurologist know he needed something else. To my mind, and likely his own, that meant a different prescription.

This "medical model"—in contrast to a more holistic approach—has undoubtedly permeated the world of primary care (and various subspecialties), where patients with multiple and/or complex problems are squeezed into fifteen-minute appointments mainly in the services of efficiency and commerce. And while this method probably works just fine for healthier people, the data increasingly shows that it doesn't do nearly as well for their sicker counterparts. The US fares poorly against other wealthier countries across a wide swath of general health measures, and one of patients' most common complaints is that doctors spend too little time with them and don't really listen to their concerns.

Doctors are dissatisfied too. More and more stories of physician burnout, depression, and substance misuse enter the public space each year, their criticisms pointing to a culture of medicine that seemingly interferes at every turn with the ancient foundation of medicine that attracted many to the field: a doctor-patient relationship in the service of bettering another's life. Some doctors have opted out of the traditional system altogether, opening concierge practices that enable them to practice closer to their ideal. Others have quit. Given the personal and institutional investment in training to become a doctor, coupled with the real shortages of physicians in many areas of the US, this is a tragedy of sorts.

In this world of physicians, psychiatrists have long occupied one of the lower rungs.

Faced with long-standing criticism, heightened perhaps to its apex in the 1960s and 1970s, for the last several decades our specialty has steadily staked its legitimacy on centering us firmly within mainstream medicine—biological, pharmacological, and technological. There is certainly an important role for all these things, yet in trying so hard to emulate internists, surgeons, and other doctors who themselves struggle under the weight of the "medical model," perhaps this validation we crave has come at the expense of our patients. And ourselves.

ERICA RETURNED TO MY OFFICE TWO WEEKS LATER. "I DON'T FEEL worse," she told me. "But I don't really feel any better either."

At our first visit, I'd taken her off two mood stabilizer drugs and a prescription sedative (she'd already stopped the antipsychotic pill) and replaced them with a single antidepressant medicine and an over-the-counter sleeping pill. She told me she didn't feel that she'd experienced any sort of withdrawal symptoms and that the new medication hadn't caused her any side effects, which to me meant that she could probably stay at the same dose a while longer. We quickly shifted from talking about medicines and symptoms as she began to discuss her life.

"I really thought things would have turned out a lot different for me," she began.

That sounded like the sort of thing one discussed with a therapist, and my first instinct was to contain the conversation and make that referral. Then, I reminded myself that we'd already agreed I would serve in that therapist role, my limitations be damned.

"What do you mean?" I asked her.

She looked at me a few seconds before speaking, her dark brown eyes tearing such that they'd soon have a red background. She told me about the two miscarriages she'd had in her early thirties. How this led to her divorce at thirty-five. And now, at thirty-nine, she'd concluded that she was never going to have a family of her own the way that her mom and sister did. Her dad's death had made those other losses more painful.

"I should be able to talk about him by now," she said haltingly, after she wiped tears and blew her nose, "without breaking down. It's not like I'm a small kid or something."

I wondered where she'd gotten her beliefs about the grief process? From her mom? Her sister? Friends? Church? Pop culture? She couldn't give me an answer.

I told her that recovering from grief wasn't necessarily a straight line from acute sorrow to "bouncing back" and that, for some people, perhaps many, setbacks could happen along the way. She looked at me skeptically at first. "Are you sure?"

I didn't have hard evidence at my disposal, but I'd heard a few chaplains and other grief counselors say as much, and I'd seen it with three or four of my patients who'd lost close relatives to suicide. As our appointment ended, she seemed a bit more relieved.

She returned again in another three weeks and began by saying that she felt better. She'd been on the antidepressant medication for nearly six weeks by then, so she was in the range when many people began to notice benefit. Before I could even think to attribute the change to pharmacology alone, she brought up what I might previously have referred to, perhaps a bit dismissively, as "therapy stuff."

"My mom and I had a long talk. We had a lot of misunderstanding."

As her dad's health progressively declined, Erica saw the mental and physical toll that it took on her mom, who had promised him she would never put him into a nursing home. Things got much worse after a debilitating stroke. A few months later, he had a severe heart attack that put him in the intensive care unit, unconscious, and barely surviving.

"After a time," Erica said, "the doctors told us he wasn't going to wake up and that they recommended we take him off life support. My mom and sister wanted to keep it going, and they argued with the doctors, but I sided with the doctors. Eventually, my mom came around to agreeing with them too. But it was really hard for her."

I thought back to various times I'd been witness to those tensions between medical teams and family members. At its worst, medical teams castigated family members as ignorant and selfish while these relatives in turn saw the white-coated staff as cruel, heartless, and, sometimes, racist.

"My mom said she doesn't blame me for agreeing with the doctors and pushing her to stop life support," Erica said as she teared up. "That she knows he was already gone and the machine was just making it seem like he was alive."

Erica hadn't just been grieving the death of her father that previous year but also carried the extra burden that she had somehow been at least partially responsible. Finding a way to move beyond that was going to take a lot longer than what could be accomplished in this thirty-minute appointment.

I saw Erica for several visits over the next six months, as she continued to make peace with her family, and herself. One day, she told me she wanted to stop the antidepressant. "I'm feeling a lot better," she said. "I'd like to see how I can do without it."

Psychiatrists probably see more people than other doctors who want to stop their medications, due to stigma around mental illness itself and, in the case of certain drugs, the real side effects that they can cause. In Erica's case, she'd made progress with her life in the interim, and a trial off meds seemed perfectly reasonable. I'd done something similar in terms of managing my high blood pressure, taking medication for many months until my diet and other lifestyle components improved enough that I could maintain a normal blood pressure without the prescription.

Our experiment failed, though, at least partially. Within three months, Erica felt she was backsliding both with an exercise program she'd started and with her productivity at work.

"Does that mean there is something wrong with me?" she asked. "With my brain?"

During my medical training, I probably would have seen it mainly through that biological lens and offered an explanation that invoked bio-chemical pathways and electrical circuitry. In that moment, however, that sort of talk felt like it would have invalidated all the efforts Erica had made to improve her psychological well-being.

"Taking the medicine again wouldn't mean you are a failure," I said, "or that you're broken in some way. Depression, grief, whatever we've been calling this, can have a lot of causes and may never go away completely. But I think you've made a lot of great strides."

"Is this a curse of being a woman?" she asked. "You know, our hormones and stuff?"

Many scientists feel that hormonal differences around menstruation, pregnancy (and postpartum), and menopause account for the higher rates of depression seen in women. Others ascribe these differences to social factors, such as gender dynamics, higher rates of physical and sexual abuse, and a greater likelihood of women seeking medical care. Simply put, all-encompassing explanations for the gender discrepancy remain elusive.

Ultimately, Erica went back on the medicine, and her mood and social engagement bounced back. She got a job promotion and started dating someone she really liked. Had restarting the antidepressant medicine produced as-yet unmeasurable changes to her brain that accounted for her better mood? Or had our continued work of psychotherapy, and what she'd done on her own to become more physically active, been the impetus for her dramatic improvement compared with our initial meeting? Or was it both? These are the sort of questions that neither biological nor psychological science can definitively answer. At least not for the foreseeable future. But that doesn't mean we can't help people in the meantime. In Erica's case, medication in the context of a good doctor-patient relationship worked best.

A year later, when Erica no longer saw me, I ran into Dr. Wang one morning in the staff break room area. She'd been the primary care doctor who had initially referred Erica to me.

"I saw your lady this morning," she said to me, referring to Erica by her last name.

My shoulders slumped. I assumed this meant she'd gotten worse. "How was she?"

Dr. Wang sipped from her large mug of coffee. "Really good," she said. "She's gotten engaged, and everything seems to be going well."

I sighed, relieved.

"Good job, Dr. Tweedy," Dr. Wang continued. "You guys do help some people."

"Same back to you," I said with equal sarcasm. "One of your patients I saw last week, Mr. Lincoln, said you've really helped him get healthy. He told me that you really listened to him a lot more than his previous doctors had."

"Go figure," Dr. Wang said, genuinely surprised. "Guess I could be a psychiatrist too."

We both laughed. We soon parted company, back to our busy daily clinic schedules. Most of the patients we would see in the days, weeks, and months ahead would not have such tidy outcomes as Erica or Mr. Lincoln, as they continued to struggle with an array of physical and emotional afflictions. And the medical system, both in how it had educated us and how it required us to practice, did us no favors in meeting these needs. Still, for me, working with Erica and being part of her transformation had shown that all was not lost. That beyond a checklist of symptoms and a prescription to minimize them, healing—whether for depression or headaches—could sometimes come from without, and within. That truth, it seemed, offered an approach to psychiatry, and to medical practice more broadly, worth doing.

He smiled, the creases prominent across his ruddy forehead and around his eyes, his teeth a few shades closer to yellow than white.

"To your question about my chest, sometimes it feels a little tight when I'm in the yard, you know, laying out mulch, but I don't really pay it much mind. Somethin' wrong?"

"How long have you noticed it, the tightness?"

It had been six weeks since his visit to his primary care physician, whose note made no mention of Doug having chest pain, tightness, or other discomfort.

"I don't know," he said. "A long time. It sort of comes and goes."

I sighed inwardly. Didn't everyone over the age of, say, fifty know that chest pain could be a sign of a heart problem and that a lot of folks died from heart attacks? But "pain" meant different things to different people. I fought back the instinct to judge him using my own medical frame of reference. I suspected that sort of condescension happened often when well-to-do white doctors interacted with their lesser-educated black patients, only I was now doing the same thing with the racial roles reversed.

"Did you tell Dr. Cohen about this?" I asked.

"It's not a new thing, like I said. When it first came up, about three or four years ago, they did a stress test on me, and they said everything was fine with my heart. What I've been feeling hasn't really felt much different from that, so I didn't even think to mention it."

I asked whether he'd had any dizziness or trouble breathing, along with an assortment of other medical-sounding questions he hadn't expected from a psychiatrist. Once I felt assured that he was safe to go home heartwise, I told him my recommendations.

"I think we can switch you back on citalopram," I said. "And I'm going to talk with Dr. Cohen about your chest tightness and your ECG."

"Thanks, Doc," he said as he shook my hand. "I appreciate you being thorough."

I saw another seven or eight patients the rest of the day, a mix of people who'd been diagnosed with PTSD, alcohol use problems, and depression, each of them mostly stable. In between visits, I thought about Doug's

9

INTEGRATION

AS I SKIMMED THE ELECTRICAL TRACING OF DOUG'S HEART, I KNEW something wasn't right. Moments earlier, Angie, a nurse at our mental health clinic, had knocked on my office door and handed me the printout of his electrocardiogram (ECG), a series of squiggly black lines with peaks and valleys set atop glossy graphing paper with a reddish background. During medical school and the first half of my intern year, I thought I'd make my living analyzing ECGs and other cardiac tests. But now, nearly a decade after switching to psychiatry, those days felt like a lifetime ago.

"Can he leave?" she asked me.

I'd finished interviewing Doug a few minutes earlier and decided at the end to get an ECG to help me decide on which medicine to prescribe him.

"Hold on a second," I said as I squinted at the black marks on the page.

Our clinic had a policy that the ordering doctor had to review the ECG before the patient could leave the clinic, to make sure something life-threatening didn't get missed.

"I have some reading glasses in my bag," she quipped. "Want me to go get them?"

I could see just fine; the problem was what was missing on the page. Normally, the ECG report spit out a series of numbers based on the arrangement of the three "waves" it measured, as well as its preliminary interpretation of whether the results were "normal" or "abnormal." For a few weeks, though, our machine had been working at half capacity, producing the usual wavy lines, but no numerical data or accompanying analysis. It felt like highway driving without the rumble strips to keep you from swerving off the road.

"When are they going to fix this thing?" I asked Angie.

"Someone is supposed to come out later this week to see if it can be repaired or if we need a new one," she replied.

Given how infrequently we ordered ECGs in psychiatry clinic, I suspected this service request ranked low on the list of medical center priorities. Without the added computerized input, that meant going back and reviewing the ECG the old-fashioned way, like I'd learned in medical school. I started with the basics. His heart rate was normal. The rhythm was normal too—no skipped beats or other irregularities. In fact, everything pretty much looked fine except one small part where the lines seemed to dip slightly when they should have been flat or trended upward. I couldn't release him to go home just yet.

"Tell him I'll be out to talk to him in a few minutes," I told Angie.

"Sure thing," she said. "Let me know if you need anything else."

The next step, if possible, was for me to find a previous ECG in the imaging section of our electronic system, to determine whether the printout showed recent changes or if the electrical activity in his heart had been stable for years. This part of our medical records was notorious for its glitches, with successful access to it a fifty-fifty proposition. On this day, I apparently called tails when I should have picked heads.

"Damn," I said aloud. "This program sucks."

I went to the waiting area to get Doug. He sat at the edge of his chair, his right leg and foot moving rhythmically up and down, his arms folded across his chest, partially covering the Carolina Hurricanes logo on his sweatshirt. He stood as I approached.

"So are we good for me to go back on my old medicine?" he asked.

Doug had started care at the VA system recently after his private family doctor retired. He'd been taking the medication citalopram for

several years and found it helpful to keep him more settled, as he described it, less anxious and irritable. But a notice from the Food and Drug Administration advised lower maximum doses of this medicine, especially in those over sixty, due to concerns about the increased risk for dangerous heart rhythm disturbances. Both advisories impacted Doug, who'd recently turned sixty-one and had been taking the highest dose. Dr. Cohen, his primary doctor in our system, switched him to a similar drug without the same risks, but it didn't seem to work. Ultimately, Doug didn't want any mental health treatment other than restarting his old medication.

"Most likely, you can," I said. "But I need to ask you some questions about your ECG. Can you come back with me for a few more minutes?"

Once back in my office, I looked at the ECG and knew where I had to start my questions.

"Have you been having any chest pain or chest tightness recently?"

Doug ran his fingers, stained and coarse from his work as a mechanic, through his still-thick, mostly gray hair. He eyed me curiously. "You said you're a psychologist, right?"

We'd sifted through this dialogue at the outset of our appointment; I'd explained that the main difference between a psychologist and psychiatrist was that I had gone to medical school and could prescribe drugs like other physicians. Some psychiatrists would have seen this need for clarification a slight, given our struggles to be seen as legitimate medical doctors, but I didn't understand the distinction myself until I was in college and began thinking about medical school. Sometimes I actually envied the greater level of psychotherapy-focused training that psychologists had in comparison. In contrast, all the years I'd spent studying microbiology, cell biology, and human anatomy seemed mostly useless when confronted with a crying patient.

"Psychiatrist," I corrected him.

"Psychiatrist," he said slowly, as if finally grasping the terminology. "That's right. I guess I didn't expect to come to see a psychiatrist and get all these medical questions."

"It's probably not how you might have seen it on TV," I replied.

ECG coupled with his chest discomfort. After my last appointment, I sped over to the primary care clinic, a fifteen-minute drive.

"Hey, Dr. Tweedy," a woman said to me from behind the front desk check-in area. "What brings you back here?"

For many years, those of us on the mental health side worked in the same office building with primary care doctors, on the opposite wing. But a few years earlier, we'd moved to a new location, desperate for additional office space. The Iraq and Afghanistan military conflicts had created a rapidly-growing veteran population nationwide, and the temperate climate and relatively affordable lifestyle in North Carolina brought transplants from all over the country, especially northeastern and midwestern states.

I spent the next few minutes chatting with the scheduling assistant and one of the clinic nurses, catching up on our lives. I then headed to Dr. Cohen's office. He was examining a stack of paper charts that had been faxed to him from a nearby hospital, his eyes desperate for rest. His curly hair had more strands of gray than when I'd last seen him many months before.

"How's it going?" I said to him. "Got a few minutes to discuss a patient?"

"Hey," he said, slapping his right hand on his knee as if trying to wake himself. "If you came all the way over from the other clinic to see me, that can't be good."

At times, it felt like we'd all been conditioned during our residency years, no matter the specialty we chose or the hospital we staffed, to anticipate the worst every time someone approached us about a patient.

"It shouldn't take long," I said. "It's about a patient of yours I saw this morning."

I showed him the ECG and summarized Doug's account of chest discomfort with physical activity.

"Why did you order it again?" Dr. Cohen asked.

"He wants to go back on citalopram. You took him off it because of the FDA advisory about QT prolongation."

"Oh yeah. I remember that. He's a good guy, but he wasn't happy with me when I switched his meds."

Citalopram and sertraline, the medicine he'd been switched to, were biochemically very similar. Yet one worked well for him while the other didn't at all. I'd seen the same happen in reverse with patients too. Why? It was one of the many mysteries that made medical practice both fascinating and frustrating.

"This does look a little funky," Dr. Cohen said as he looked at the ECG. "Does he have an old one to compare?"

"I'm not sure. I couldn't get the imaging program to work."

"Let's see if it likes me any better."

It did. After a few mouse clicks, Dr. Cohen had pulled up an ECG done a few years earlier when Doug came to the ER with abdominal pain.

"Well, well, well," Dr. Cohen said as he compared the two tracings.

The first ECG was essentially normal. The one I'd ordered that morning clearly wasn't, suggesting something with his heart had changed in the interim.

"He's got ST depressions in his inferior leads," Dr. Cohen said. "And that lines up with the exertional ischemia you described."

In plain terms, this meant that a portion of Doug's heart wasn't getting the oxygen it needed, likely due to a blockage in one of his arteries. Earlier in my training, this medical jargon had been part of my regular work, and I found myself enjoying the change of pace from my current daily talk of suicide, insomnia, and excessive drinking.

Dr. Cohen switched back to the main medical record file, and pulled up the notes he'd written after seeing Doug. "He never said anything about chest pain. I always ask about that. Why wouldn't he tell me?"

I relayed Doug's description of having had the same discomfort years earlier followed by a normal cardiac stress test.

"Interesting," he said. "Well, this time around, he's bought himself a referral to the cardiology clinic, and I suspect they're going to do more than just a stress test."

"Will you call him and explain things to him?" I asked. "Or do you want me to?"

"I'll take it from here," he said as a smile spread across his face. "Very good work, Dr. Tweedy. I wasn't due to see him for another six months.

Who knows what could have happened between now and then? You very well just might have saved this guy's life."

After Dr. Cohen entered the electronic referral to the cardiology team, we spent the next several minutes chatting. We commiserated over the challenges of our work. This exchange reminded us of how much overlap we shared, despite the divides—both literal and metaphorical—between our medical specialties. People with physical problems were prone to emotional suffering, and those whose issues we deemed psychological inhabited physical bodies in need of care. It was an undeniable truth, yet roadblocks and minefields littered this mind-body landscape.

As family responsibilities demanded we go our separate ways, Dr. Cohen and I remarked on how good it was to see each other again. What should have been a regular occurrence was in fact something that happened less and less frequently with doctors as our medical careers progressed, to the detriment of our patients. And to us.

THERE ARE CERTAIN AREAS OF HEALTH CARE WHERE THE WORK OF physicians, at its best, operates seamlessly in tandem. The colon polyp removed by the gastroenterologist is analyzed by the pathologist for signs of cancer. The family physician or gynecologist orders a mammogram read by the radiologist. An obstetrician hands over a premature newborn to a specialty pediatrician (neonatologist). And in these and other encounters, the doctors work in concert with nurses, physician assistants, physical therapists, clinical pharmacists, and various other health care providers.

All this good collegiality happens a lot less often when we're dealing with emotional problems, however. Family doctors, on average, have little difficulty getting their patients referred to see surgeons, cardiologists, or oncologists. But getting that same person to see a psychiatrist feels like the difference between running a mile versus a marathon. I saw this vividly one morning during my intern year when our team prepared to discharge a young man with type 1 diabetes we'd admitted after he overdosed on insulin. Badly confused, he'd crashed his car into a mailbox and broken his wrist.

A psychiatrist on the hospital consult service saw him and determined that the overdose was unintentional. Nonetheless, they felt he was clinically depressed and recommended outpatient care. While it took only a few minutes to arrange aftercare appointments with an endocrinologist for diabetes care and an orthopedic surgeon to treat his fracture, it took an hour to find an appointment with a psychiatrist, and what we got, in the end, was far from ideal.

Many of the psychiatry offices I called didn't answer the phone. Those who did said that they weren't taking on new patients or, if they were, that they didn't accept health insurance payments, meaning the patient had to pay the full price of the visit. Psychiatrists, as it turns out, are least likely among doctors to accept health insurance. This is partly because reimbursement isn't on par with general medicine payments, and also because in many larger population areas, the market for their services allows them to prosper without the need to deal with the hassles and constraints health insurers place upon them. For this patient, that meant that while he could visit high-quality physicians in the Raleigh area for his diabetes and his wrist fracture, to see a psychiatrist, the best I could get him was a forty-five-minute drive to see a second-year psychiatry resident learning the ropes of clinical practice. In addition to the larger stigma in seeking mental health treatment, these added barriers were a recipe for this patient, and others like him, to simply stay home.

The chasm between psychiatry and general medicine became even more evident when I switched to psychiatry and saw things from the other side. Sometimes this disconnect wasn't simply about the logistics of making referrals and scheduling appointments but about the very nature of the work that we did.

A few years after residency, I found myself in an electronic back-and-forth with another doctor when the drug I prescribed for a patient with bipolar disorder interacted with the one that he ordered for an autoimmune condition. Neither of us wanted to budge, given the risk that switching to another drug could cause a relapse in the respective conditions we were treating. What became clear was how little each of us knew about the other's field and the various medicines that we used. We'd started

9

INTEGRATION

AS I SKIMMED THE ELECTRICAL TRACING OF DOUG'S HEART, I KNEW something wasn't right. Moments earlier, Angie, a nurse at our mental health clinic, had knocked on my office door and handed me the printout of his electrocardiogram (ECG), a series of squiggly black lines with peaks and valleys set atop glossy graphing paper with a reddish background. During medical school and the first half of my intern year, I thought I'd make my living analyzing ECGs and other cardiac tests. But now, nearly a decade after switching to psychiatry, those days felt like a lifetime ago.

"Can he leave?" she asked me.

I'd finished interviewing Doug a few minutes earlier and decided at the end to get an ECG to help me decide on which medicine to prescribe him.

"Hold on a second," I said as I squinted at the black marks on the page.

Our clinic had a policy that the ordering doctor had to review the ECG before the patient could leave the clinic, to make sure something life-threatening didn't get missed.

"I have some reading glasses in my bag," she quipped. "Want me to go get them?"

I could see just fine; the problem was what was missing on the page. Normally, the ECG report spit out a series of numbers based on the arrangement of the three "waves" it measured, as well as its preliminary interpretation of whether the results were "normal" or "abnormal." For a few weeks, though, our machine had been working at half capacity, producing the usual wavy lines, but no numerical data or accompanying analysis. It felt like highway driving without the rumble strips to keep you from swerving off the road.

"When are they going to fix this thing?" I asked Angie.

"Someone is supposed to come out later this week to see if it can be repaired or if we need a new one," she replied.

Given how infrequently we ordered ECGs in psychiatry clinic, I suspected this service request ranked low on the list of medical center priorities. Without the added computerized input, that meant going back and reviewing the ECG the old-fashioned way, like I'd learned in medical school. I started with the basics. His heart rate was normal. The rhythm was normal too—no skipped beats or other irregularities. In fact, everything pretty much looked fine except one small part where the lines seemed to dip slightly when they should have been flat or trended upward. I couldn't release him to go home just yet.

"Tell him I'll be out to talk to him in a few minutes," I told Angie.

"Sure thing," she said. "Let me know if you need anything else."

The next step, if possible, was for me to find a previous ECG in the imaging section of our electronic system, to determine whether the printout showed recent changes or if the electrical activity in his heart had been stable for years. This part of our medical records was notorious for its glitches, with successful access to it a fifty-fifty proposition. On this day, I apparently called tails when I should have picked heads.

"Damn," I said aloud. "This program sucks."

I went to the waiting area to get Doug. He sat at the edge of his chair, his right leg and foot moving rhythmically up and down, his arms folded across his chest, partially covering the Carolina Hurricanes logo on his sweatshirt. He stood as I approached.

"So are we good for me to go back on my old medicine?" he asked.

Doug had started care at the VA system recently after his private family doctor retired. He'd been taking the medication citalopram for several years and found it helpful to keep him more settled, as he described it, less anxious and irritable. But a notice from the Food and Drug Administration advised lower maximum doses of this medicine, especially in those over sixty, due to concerns about the increased risk for dangerous heart rhythm disturbances. Both advisories impacted Doug, who'd recently turned sixty-one and had been taking the highest dose. Dr. Cohen, his primary doctor in our system, switched him to a similar drug without the same risks, but it didn't seem to work. Ultimately, Doug didn't want any mental health treatment other than restarting his old medication.

"Most likely, you can," I said. "But I need to ask you some questions about your ECG. Can you come back with me for a few more minutes?"

Once back in my office, I looked at the ECG and knew where I had to start my questions.

"Have you been having any chest pain or chest tightness recently?"

Doug ran his fingers, stained and coarse from his work as a mechanic, through his still-thick, mostly gray hair. He eyed me curiously. "You said you're a psychologist, right?"

We'd sifted through this dialogue at the outset of our appointment; I'd explained that the main difference between a psychologist and psychiatrist was that I had gone to medical school and could prescribe drugs like other physicians. Some psychiatrists would have seen this need for clarification a slight, given our struggles to be seen as legitimate medical doctors, but I didn't understand the distinction myself until I was in college and began thinking about medical school. Sometimes I actually envied the greater level of psychotherapy-focused training that psychologists had in comparison. In contrast, all the years I'd spent studying microbiology, cell biology, and human anatomy seemed mostly useless when confronted with a crying patient.

"Psychiatrist," I corrected him.

"Psychiatrist," he said slowly, as if finally grasping the terminology. "That's right. I guess I didn't expect to come to see a psychiatrist and get all these medical questions."

"It's probably not how you might have seen it on TV," I replied.

He smiled, the creases prominent across his ruddy forehead and around his eyes, his teeth a few shades closer to yellow than white.

"To your question about my chest, sometimes it feels a little tight when I'm in the yard, you know, laying out mulch, but I don't really pay it much mind. Somethin' wrong?"

"How long have you noticed it, the tightness?"

It had been six weeks since his visit to his primary care physician, whose note made no mention of Doug having chest pain, tightness, or other discomfort.

"I don't know," he said. "A long time. It sort of comes and goes."

I sighed inwardly. Didn't everyone over the age of, say, fifty know that chest pain could be a sign of a heart problem and that a lot of folks died from heart attacks? But "pain" meant different things to different people. I fought back the instinct to judge him using my own medical frame of reference. I suspected that sort of condescension happened often when well-to-do white doctors interacted with their lesser-educated black patients, only I was now doing the same thing with the racial roles reversed.

"Did you tell Dr. Cohen about this?" I asked.

"It's not a new thing, like I said. When it first came up, about three or four years ago, they did a stress test on me, and they said everything was fine with my heart. What I've been feeling hasn't really felt much different from that, so I didn't even think to mention it."

I asked whether he'd had any dizziness or trouble breathing, along with an assortment of other medical-sounding questions he hadn't expected from a psychiatrist. Once I felt assured that he was safe to go home heartwise, I told him my recommendations.

"I think we can switch you back on citalopram," I said. "And I'm going to talk with Dr. Cohen about your chest tightness and your ECG."

"Thanks, Doc," he said as he shook my hand. "I appreciate you being thorough."

I saw another seven or eight patients the rest of the day, a mix of people who'd been diagnosed with PTSD, alcohol use problems, and depression, each of them mostly stable. In between visits, I thought about Doug's

ECG coupled with his chest discomfort. After my last appointment, I sped over to the primary care clinic, a fifteen-minute drive.

"Hey, Dr. Tweedy," a woman said to me from behind the front desk check-in area. "What brings you back here?"

For many years, those of us on the mental health side worked in the same office building with primary care doctors, on the opposite wing. But a few years earlier, we'd moved to a new location, desperate for additional office space. The Iraq and Afghanistan military conflicts had created a rapidly-growing veteran population nationwide, and the temperate climate and relatively affordable lifestyle in North Carolina brought transplants from all over the country, especially northeastern and midwestern states.

I spent the next few minutes chatting with the scheduling assistant and one of the clinic nurses, catching up on our lives. I then headed to Dr. Cohen's office. He was examining a stack of paper charts that had been faxed to him from a nearby hospital, his eyes desperate for rest. His curly hair had more strands of gray than when I'd last seen him many months before.

"How's it going?" I said to him. "Got a few minutes to discuss a patient?"

"Hey," he said, slapping his right hand on his knee as if trying to wake himself. "If you came all the way over from the other clinic to see me, that can't be good."

At times, it felt like we'd all been conditioned during our residency years, no matter the specialty we chose or the hospital we staffed, to anticipate the worst every time someone approached us about a patient.

"It shouldn't take long," I said. "It's about a patient of yours I saw this morning."

I showed him the ECG and summarized Doug's account of chest discomfort with physical activity.

"Why did you order it again?" Dr. Cohen asked.

"He wants to go back on citalopram. You took him off it because of the FDA advisory about QT prolongation."

"Oh yeah. I remember that. He's a good guy, but he wasn't happy with me when I switched his meds."

Citalopram and sertraline, the medicine he'd been switched to, were biochemically very similar. Yet one worked well for him while the other didn't at all. I'd seen the same happen in reverse with patients too. Why? It was one of the many mysteries that made medical practice both fascinating and frustrating.

"This does look a little funky," Dr. Cohen said as he looked at the ECG. "Does he have an old one to compare?"

"I'm not sure. I couldn't get the imaging program to work."

"Let's see if it likes me any better."

It did. After a few mouse clicks, Dr. Cohen had pulled up an ECG done a few years earlier when Doug came to the ER with abdominal pain.

"Well, well, well," Dr. Cohen said as he compared the two tracings.

The first ECG was essentially normal. The one I'd ordered that morning clearly wasn't, suggesting something with his heart had changed in the interim.

"He's got ST depressions in his inferior leads," Dr. Cohen said. "And that lines up with the exertional ischemia you described."

In plain terms, this meant that a portion of Doug's heart wasn't getting the oxygen it needed, likely due to a blockage in one of his arteries. Earlier in my training, this medical jargon had been part of my regular work, and I found myself enjoying the change of pace from my current daily talk of suicide, insomnia, and excessive drinking.

Dr. Cohen switched back to the main medical record file, and pulled up the notes he'd written after seeing Doug. "He never said anything about chest pain. I always ask about that. Why wouldn't he tell me?"

I relayed Doug's description of having had the same discomfort years earlier followed by a normal cardiac stress test.

"Interesting," he said. "Well, this time around, he's bought himself a referral to the cardiology clinic, and I suspect they're going to do more than just a stress test."

"Will you call him and explain things to him?" I asked. "Or do you want me to?"

"I'll take it from here," he said as a smile spread across his face. "Very good work, Dr. Tweedy. I wasn't due to see him for another six months.

Who knows what could have happened between now and then? You very well just might have saved this guy's life."

After Dr. Cohen entered the electronic referral to the cardiology team, we spent the next several minutes chatting. We commiserated over the challenges of our work. This exchange reminded us of how much overlap we shared, despite the divides—both literal and metaphorical—between our medical specialties. People with physical problems were prone to emotional suffering, and those whose issues we deemed psychological inhabited physical bodies in need of care. It was an undeniable truth, yet roadblocks and minefields littered this mind-body landscape.

As family responsibilities demanded we go our separate ways, Dr. Cohen and I remarked on how good it was to see each other again. What should have been a regular occurrence was in fact something that happened less and less frequently with doctors as our medical careers progressed, to the detriment of our patients. And to us.

THERE ARE CERTAIN AREAS OF HEALTH CARE WHERE THE WORK OF physicians, at its best, operates seamlessly in tandem. The colon polyp removed by the gastroenterologist is analyzed by the pathologist for signs of cancer. The family physician or gynecologist orders a mammogram read by the radiologist. An obstetrician hands over a premature newborn to a specialty pediatrician (neonatologist). And in these and other encounters, the doctors work in concert with nurses, physician assistants, physical therapists, clinical pharmacists, and various other health care providers.

All this good collegiality happens a lot less often when we're dealing with emotional problems, however. Family doctors, on average, have little difficulty getting their patients referred to see surgeons, cardiologists, or oncologists. But getting that same person to see a psychiatrist feels like the difference between running a mile versus a marathon. I saw this vividly one morning during my intern year when our team prepared to discharge a young man with type 1 diabetes we'd admitted after he overdosed on insulin. Badly confused, he'd crashed his car into a mailbox and broken his wrist.

A psychiatrist on the hospital consult service saw him and determined that the overdose was unintentional. Nonetheless, they felt he was clinically depressed and recommended outpatient care. While it took only a few minutes to arrange aftercare appointments with an endocrinologist for diabetes care and an orthopedic surgeon to treat his fracture, it took an hour to find an appointment with a psychiatrist, and what we got, in the end, was far from ideal.

Many of the psychiatry offices I called didn't answer the phone. Those who did said that they weren't taking on new patients or, if they were, that they didn't accept health insurance payments, meaning the patient had to pay the full price of the visit. Psychiatrists, as it turns out, are least likely among doctors to accept health insurance. This is partly because reimbursement isn't on par with general medicine payments, and also because in many larger population areas, the market for their services allows them to prosper without the need to deal with the hassles and constraints health insurers place upon them. For this patient, that meant that while he could visit high-quality physicians in the Raleigh area for his diabetes and his wrist fracture, to see a psychiatrist, the best I could get him was a forty-five-minute drive to see a second-year psychiatry resident learning the ropes of clinical practice. In addition to the larger stigma in seeking mental health treatment, these added barriers were a recipe for this patient, and others like him, to simply stay home.

The chasm between psychiatry and general medicine became even more evident when I switched to psychiatry and saw things from the other side. Sometimes this disconnect wasn't simply about the logistics of making referrals and scheduling appointments but about the very nature of the work that we did.

A few years after residency, I found myself in an electronic back-and-forth with another doctor when the drug I prescribed for a patient with bipolar disorder interacted with the one that he ordered for an autoimmune condition. Neither of us wanted to budge, given the risk that switching to another drug could cause a relapse in the respective conditions we were treating. What became clear was how little each of us knew about the other's field and the various medicines that we used. We'd started out in the same lecture halls and clinical laboratories as newbie student doctors, but years later, we'd come to speak entirely different languages. It took the efforts of a wonderful clinical pharmacist—part translator, part mediator—to break the gridlock and find a workable solution for our patient.

When I met Doug, I'd been on staff at the outpatient clinic for over five years and had become ensconced in the mental health world. My everyday colleagues were social workers, psychologists, and other psychiatrists, not gynecologists, dermatologists, and neurologists. Sitting in an office several highway exits away from the primary care building, I found myself increasingly detached from the challenges these doctors faced too, more critical of the volume of patients they sent our way, and of how little information their referrals to us usually contained. I had come to see them as adversaries, blinded to the challenges they faced, ones I recently discussed with Dr. Danielle Ofri, a celebrated writer and primary care doctor at Bellevue Hospital in New York City.

"Nearly every single patient I see in the medical clinic has mental health concerns mixed with everything else," she told me. "Depression, stress, and anxiety percolate through people's lives and affect everything from their adherence to medications, their ability to exercise, their bandwidth to prepare healthy food over grabbing McDonald's, and their capacity to focus on their other illnesses."

Viewed that way, Ofri and other primary care doctors are doing much of the heavy lifting addressing their patients' emotional problems. But at the time, I could see only my side and how overwhelmed I often felt with the referrals they sent us.

My thinking might have continued this way had it not been for the morning I opened our electronic record system and saw a note addressed to several psychiatrists at our clinic. A primary care doctor pleaded with us to call a patient of hers who was a military contractor with a security clearance that he feared losing if his medical record indicated any visits to the mental health clinic. He was having trouble sleeping and experiencing distressing recollections about his time in Iraq but had refused to do more than talk with her about these issues for twenty minutes every three months. She didn't feel qualified to handle his concerns and worried that he would spiral further downward.

I soon came to realize that for each referral sent our way, general practice providers managed others who refused our services because of the stigma they attached to mental illness or the repercussions they feared awaited them if their visit to a psychiatrist or other mental health practitioner became known to others. And many more patients, especially in the world outside the VA health system, simply couldn't afford the cost of a therapist. That left primary care doctors to bear the brunt of their patients' emotional struggles, working within a system poorly suited to addressing those needs.

"If I had an hour for each patient, I could probably provide reasonable mental health care for most of my patients," Dr. Ofri said, "but I have fifteen minutes and often can't even make it through all of their other medical issues."

What patients needed was something our hospital system had devised in theory but not yet employed in practice: access to mental health providers at the time of a general medical visit. Someone who could quickly triage mental illness concerns and devise a workable plan for the patient. Leadership agreed. That person—along with a team of staff operating in the same capacity—ended up being me. Early in my tenure, less than a year after meeting Doug, I saw an older man who cemented for me the lifesaving potential of this approach to care.

WILLIE HAD BEEN THINKING ABOUT KILLING HIMSELF FOR WEEKS. But I wouldn't know that, or how close he came to doing so, until much later. In retrospect, maybe that was best.

We met on a Friday morning when a primary care nurse escorted him from the other side of the building into my office. He looked back at her, hesitant.

"This is Dr. Tweedy," she said to him as she smiled. "Our psychiatrist."

A few months earlier, our hospital had been given a mandate to more fully integrate behavioral health services into our primary care clinics.

Before that, on a part-time basis, I'd led a small team of mental health nurses who followed, a few dozen at a time, patients taking antidepressants. But that was no longer sufficient. Along with funds to hire more staff—two psychologists, a social worker, and a nurse practitioner—came expectations that we would be available to see patients in a warm-handoff format, immediately after primary care visits. Fridays were my day to staff this particular clinic.

Because it was Willie's annual primary care visit, a nurse at the clinic had asked him two questions about his mood; based on his responses, the results were "positive," and his primary care physician was alerted. She then asked him a few more questions and decided it was time to try out our new same-day access service. I picked up from there.

"My life ain't no good," Willie said to me as he looked at my shoes, my slacks, my dress shirt and tie, seemingly inspecting me with curiosity. "But I'd like to hear about yours. Where'd you get your education at?"

Sometimes when patients—black, white, or otherwise—asked about my credentials, I wondered if they felt that I, as a black man, was somehow a less legitimate doctor.

"I went to medical school at Duke," I said, hoping he'd stop his inquiries there.

His eyes widened through his thick glasses as he repositioned his body in the chair, trying to make himself more comfortable. He rubbed his scalp, which was mostly bald.

"Duke. Look at you. Man, you know when I was young, that place didn't even allow black folks on campus unless they were there to clean up after those rich white folks."

I'd heard many versions of that story over the years. Duke University as we know it was established in 1924 and, in keeping with the traditions of the Jim Crow era, remained segregated into the early 1960s. Willie would have been eighteen or nineteen when Duke first integrated, and the sting of second-class citizenship had been something he'd experienced firsthand, as had his parents before him. His comment made me think about my parents, who were a few years older than he was, and their stories about life back then.

"I guess some things have changed," he continued as he looked off at the wall behind me. "But sometimes it don't seem much has. I see these young fools around here with their pants sagging and jacking up our own people. And I see cops wanting to beat us up with no consequences. Dr. King must be turning over in his grave."

I'd heard my parents talk that way many times, their perspective often at odds with the many young black people I knew—aspiring lawyers, dentists, and physicians who were doing just fine. Would I become so pessimistic when I got their age? I hoped not.

"Is this what has been getting you down?" I asked. "Other people's struggles?"

"Our people's struggles," he corrected me. "It's getting worse rather than better."

Willie explained how his nephew's two kids had fallen on hard times. The son was serving time in jail for a drug charge while the daughter had dropped out of college and was uncertain about her next steps. This wasn't how it was supposed to have turned out.

"My nephew was the family jewel," he explained. "All-state tennis. Smart as a whip. Graduated top honors from Howard."

My mom's voice echoed in my head. She spoke with dismay about coworkers, cousins, and other working- and middle-class black people whose children had seemingly slid down the prosperity ladder. Each generation of black folks was supposed to build upon the gains made by the previous one. We'd struggled through too much to give it all away.

"Do you have children yourself?" I asked Willie. "Grandchildren?"

"No," he said as his eyes met mine briefly. "My wife and I didn't get married until our late thirties, and it just didn't work out. We made peace with that a long time ago."

Willie told me that he'd retired from a mid-level corporate job two years earlier and that he and his wife had traveled quite a bit with a church group during that first year. But then his mother-in-law broke her hip and ended up needing to move in with them. Soon after, the trips stopped. He suddenly had a lot more time at home, and was unsure how to spend it.

From there, I transitioned to a typical psychiatric interview. Willie didn't have any previous encounters with a mental health professional. Nothing raised alarms as far as him misusing alcohol or other substances. Basically, he came across as a depressed older man, the kind I'd seen hundreds of times before. As always, I asked if he'd ever thought about suicide.

"That would be giving the white man what he wants, right?" he responded.

He didn't really answer the question, so I tried again and more or less got the same response. I decided that was good enough. I asked him his thoughts on next treatment steps, explaining that some people did talk therapy, others took meds, and some wanted both, or neither. We settled on him coming back in three weeks, as this new integrated model allowed more scheduling flexibility than the regular clinic.

"Thanks, my brother," he said to me. "Guess I should say *Dr. Brother.*"

We both smiled. I felt like we'd made a good doctor-patient connection, aided by our shared history as black men across two generations. He reminded me of my parents in some respects, and he told me that I reminded him of his nephew as a younger person. Psychiatrists call this *countertransference* and *transference*, respectively, but in that moment, it simply felt like good doctoring to someone who needed a boost.

That's why I was surprised when he didn't come for his follow-up visit. As possible explanations for his no-show—ranging from the benign to the morbid—rattled in my mind, I dialed his number.

Willie answered on the fourth or fifth ring, his voice faint, distant.

"This is Dr. Tweedy," I said. "We met a few weeks ago at the clinic and scheduled a follow-up appointment for this morning."

"Hey, Doc," he said as he brought the phone receiver closer to his mouth. "I wasn't feeling too good this morning. Think I got a bad cold or something. The appointment slipped my mind. Sorry about that. Hope I didn't mess up your day somehow."

"No problem," I said. "Did you want to reschedule?"

There was a long pause. The kind where someone is trying to think of how to get themselves out of a situation. Maybe Willie didn't want a second appointment but was afraid he'd come off like he was offending me.

"Or you can call me back later and we can go from there?" I said, offering him an escape.

This time, there was a shorter pause, awkward still: "When's your next opening?"

We scheduled for the following Friday, when I would be at that same clinic.

"Thanks for checking up on me, Doc," he said at the end of our call. "It's really good to hear your voice."

Willie arrived fifteen minutes early the next Friday and said he felt better, physically and mentally. The tennis US Open was on television, and that motivated him to go to a neighborhood park to hit some balls off a wooden wall. There, he stumbled upon a tennis clinic where a college-age student was teaching some small kids the basics of the sport.

"It was a beautiful thing to watch," he said.

We spent the next ten minutes talking about black professional tennis players. Althea Gibson. Arthur Ashe. The Williams sisters. And several lesser-known ones.

At the end of the visit, Willie acknowledged that he'd been depressed for some time and asked if I could write him a prescription.

"Something low-dose," he said. "I don't want to be a zombie or nothing."

Willie took only one other medicine, a pill for high blood pressure, and I sensed that making this request was a big deal for him. I complied and prescribed a common antidepressant, but at half-strength.

"So good to see you again, brother," he said as he left my office.

Willie came back the next month and seemed better. It all sounded like a breezy feel-good psychiatry story, the kind that made our work seem worthwhile in the midst of many others that didn't go nearly as well. It was only later that I learned the messier truth. On our sixth visit, many months after our first meeting, he dropped a bombshell.

"You know, Doc," he began as he rubbed his hands on his thighs. "That first day I met you. That was going to be it for me. The end."

My stomach lurched slightly. I felt a tingle in the back of my neck. "You mean . . . ?"

"Suicide. Self-murder. I had it all worked out."

My intent had been to talk to Willie about how my role in this inte-grated model was to provide short-term care and that I felt he was ready to have his primary care doctor refill his future antidepressant prescrip-tions. So much for that.

"Uh, how?" I asked.

He told me that one month before we met, he tweaked his lower back one morning mowing his lawn. A few hours later, he and his wife ar-gued, a rarity for them, and he decided that he was useless and taking up space. Just like that. But he didn't want anything messy or to leave his wife with the shame of knowing he'd killed himself.

"I came up with a plan to go fishing on my boat real early in the morning and take a bunch of sleeping pills out on the lake," he be-gan, "and then fall into the water. If someone found me, they'd think it was an accident. I saw you on a Friday and was going out there the next morning. I bought the pills a while ago, so no one would have suspected a thing."

I thought back to our first meeting, when Willie described suicide as "giv-ing the white man what he wants." He sounded defiant, yet now, it seemed, he had been lying to my face. I felt a flash of anger course through me.

"Why did you come here to see Dr. Olsen that day, then?"

Dr. Olsen was his primary doctor, the one who'd sent him to see me immediately after his appointment with her. "She's been good to me," he answered. "Her appointment was scheduled months before—you know, before I started thinking of checking out. I wanted to see her and say goodbye. But when she started talking about depression and then sent me to you, I figured maybe that was a sign from above not to end things just yet."

I squirmed in my seat. I wasn't particularly religious and struggled to believe that God had used me to intervene on Willie's behalf. That went against my rational brain. Yet had he come to see Dr. Olsen even three months earlier for his "final" visit, there would have been no same-day services; instead, she would have placed an electronic consult, and a scheduling clerk would have called him several days later to make an appointment. If that call was answered, it would have been his distraught wife informing the clerk that her husband was dead, from a boating accident that was actually suicide.

Willie told me that he still felt bad after meeting me and thought a lot about suicide. That was why he didn't show up for our second appointment.

"I don't know if I was going to go through with the plan," he said, "but I definitely wasn't going to come back to see you. I thought it would be wasting your time. I didn't expect you to call to check up on me. That was another lifeline."

Doctors are somewhat notorious for having a god complex, but I never felt that way at all. Not once. While I liked the idea of acquiring knowledge and skills to help people, the notion that I could be the most important person a patient encountered at any stage of their life never sat well with me.

"Well, I'm glad you're still here," I said honestly.

"I am too," he said, laughing as he clapped his hands together.

Rather than embrace Willie's joy in that moment, however, I found myself backtracking, wondering if I'd made a mistake in missing his earlier inner distress. His cynicism about racial progress mirrored my parents', and now I wondered if that similarity had blinded me to his despair. Could that countertransference theory stuff, which I'd mostly dismissed as weird, overly intellectual psychobabble, have been at work?

"You okay, Doc?" Willie asked.

"Sure," I said as I squeezed my hand into a fist for a second before releasing it.

He'd briefly brought me back to the moment. But not for long. As Willie talked about going to a girls' high school basketball tournament, my mind wandered to how I might have handled that initial visit had I known he was suicidal. At a minimum, I would have focused the entire visit in a more clinical, diagnostic way, with prescribing medicine my primary goal. Depending on how that went, I may have escalated things further, insisting he went to the hospital, on his own, or by way of police. Looking back, those actions might have made things worse. Still, my training and experience would have compelled me in that direction.

As the visit wound to a close, that medical impulse returned. "Right now, your dose is at half the recommended level," I said. "One option could be to bump it up some. Another option could be you seeing one of our psychologists for cognitive-behavioral therapy."

Willie smiled again. "Relax, Doc," he said. "I'm doing much better. I definitely want to stick around as long as I'm staying active and feeling like I got a reason to be here. I don't need to see anyone else or take any extra pills. I'll let you know if that changes."

I laughed nervously at the irony that our roles had reversed: the patient was now consoling the doctor. We continued talking for several more minutes as Willie went into some detail about charity work he was doing for a local Salvation Army branch leading up to Christmas. With each passing minute, my anxiety ebbed. Willie was going to be okay.

I thought again how differently it could have all turned out. My presence down the hall from Dr. Olsen had been, in Willie's words, literally lifesaving. Even had he not killed himself, the referral call from the scheduling clerk would likely have gone unanswered. They often were. Meeting Willie in the flesh, without delay, had, seemingly, been magical.

THE ARRANGEMENT IN WHICH I SAW WILLIE—RIGHT AFTER HIS PRIMARY care appointment—is part of a package of services with a name that is steadily becoming part of the medical lexicon: *collaborative care*. Developed during the 1990s, the approach arose from an indisputably problematic trifecta: vast numbers of patients relied on primary care doctors to treat their emotional distress; these physicians were poorly trained and too busy to manage this problem; and inadequately addressed mental health problems worsened physical health outcomes. Bringing mental health services into the primary care setting had the potential to revolutionize medicine.

Like most reform in the American health care arena, implementation has proven challenging. Who will pay for the startup and maintenance costs for new staff, especially in smaller medical practices? How will health insurers reimburse medical services based heavily on doctors talking to each other, rather than working alone on patients' separate body parts? What could motivate primary care doctors and psychiatrists who've trained under the traditional model of body versus mind to shift gears?

From studies conducted in varied settings and locations, the data promoting change is persuasive: collaborative care makes patients more likely to get mental health treatment, reduces the burden of depression that complicates various medical conditions such as diabetes, and improves patient and primary care provider satisfaction, all while ultimately reducing health care costs. Nonetheless, reform is hard. The vast majority of patients visiting a family physician or other similar doctor will not have the immediate assistance Willie received, whether from me, a psychologist, a clinical social worker, or other mental health worker. They'll rely on the old model, which fails many people.

In researching this book, I wanted to gain perspective on what the future could look like. I spoke about collaborative care with Dr. Frank deGruy, then chair of family medicine at the University of Colorado and a pioneer in the field. As a medical student in the 1970s, his specialty choice came down to family medicine versus psychiatry: he chose family medicine because his psychiatry rotation (like mine) seemed too narrow, focused exclusively on the most severe forms of mental illness. As a family medicine resident, though, a different exposure to psychiatry— one where he saw a broader array of people and their problems—allowed him to think about mental illness differently.

"I saw how much emotional well-being impacted health at every level," he told me.

He soon began a research career, studying how mental disorders and unexplained physical symptoms manifested and were addressed in primary care. Later, when he became a leader in academic medicine, Dr. deGruy put into practice his beliefs that good primary care always includes mental and behavioral elements. At the University of Colorado program he helped develop, the seven outpatient family medicine clinics all have embedded psychologists and social workers on staff, as well as four psychiatrists spread across the enterprise. There, the integrated staff meet people like Willie and are prepared to treat the "whole person," not just a disease or specific body part.

Despite this transformative approach to health care, deGruy does not see integrated health care as an existential threat to the existing medical order.

"There is never going to be less demand for psychiatry as a hard-core discipline delivering specialty care," he told me. "But we need a layer of psychiatry and psychology that runs through all medical disciplines, especially primary care."

Dr. deGruy led me to other leaders in this arena. Dr. Jürgen Unützer, chair of psychiatry at the University of Washington and a pioneer in implementing collaborative care from the psychiatric side, told me that "even if we somehow doubled the number of psychiatrists in private practice, we still wouldn't help a lot of people where they need this care the most, at their primary doctor's office." Dr. Parinda Khatri, a psychologist and leader of the Cherokee Health Systems in Tennessee, echoed these sentiments and added that the traditional model of outpatient psychiatry and psychology was too limiting. "You don't have to have a mental health diagnosis and receive long-term therapy," she said, "to benefit from addressing behavioral health issues that impact your overall health." Dr. Alexander Blount, a Massachusetts-based psychologist and leading educator and innovator in the field of integrated care, agreed, telling me there was plenty of blame to spread around on both sides for the status quo: "For too long, those working in general medicine and mental health have been at odds, skeptical of the other, when they should be working in tandem."

These doctors spoke passionately about their work, peppering me with examples of projects they'd helped lead to improve mental health care in general medicine settings. For Unützer, that meant training psychiatrists to supervise mental health nurses and collaborate with primary care doctors in distant locations. For Khatri, integrating behavioral medicine and primary care in her health system meant expanding beyond general adult medicine clinics and including pediatric and obstetrics settings. Blount talked about his tireless efforts to educate health care systems throughout America on ways to implement a sound integrated care model.

I left these conversations trying to imagine how different my medical

school experiences might have been with this approach. Would my only formal exposure to psychiatry have taken place in a state hospital where I witnessed patients being restrained and forcibly injected with drugs? Or might I have also had the opportunity to see people with mental afflictions doing well in the outside world? Would the patients who smoked cigarettes, drank too much alcohol, and used other drugs despite serious health consequences still have been castigated as "drug seekers" who made bad choices, or might I have been exposed to medical personnel who treated addiction compassionately and effectively? Had my medical foundation, both in general medicine and psychiatry, caused me to unwittingly harm patients over the years?

As I pondered these questions, Dr. deGruy's final words left me with a measure of hope. "When I started in this field," he told me, "people would say, 'Why do we need this?' But now people are saying, 'How do we do this?' That's real progress."

THIS "LAYER" OF MENTAL HEALTH SERVICES SURROUNDING GEN-eral medical care undoubtedly worked to improve Doug's life, if not save it altogether. A little over a year before Willie freed his mind from suicidal thinking, Doug—the man whose previous antidepressant pill had come under tighter restrictions—was relieved from the grips of his own life-threatening health problem.

"Dr. Tweedy," he said, his voice penetrating as he strode confidently into my office three months later. "The man of the hour. You saved my life."

My basketball-playing days had entrenched a focus on losses over wins, on miscues rather than good plays, and that mindset had seeped into my medical career. Still, I couldn't hold back a small smile.

"I see that the cardiologists got you all fixed up," I said.

After I had reviewed his abnormal ECG with Dr. Cohen (his primary care doctor), Doug got referred to the cardiology clinic at our hospital. Because I didn't place the request, I remained oblivious to the results until Doug returned to see me. Literally two minutes before his appointment time, I skimmed his medical chart for updates, my usual practice

whenever I got the chance. Sometimes, the patient hadn't seen anyone in the interim, visits with me their only connection to the health care system. Doug's chart, in contrast, revealed a slew of medical notes from cardiology staff. A heart catheterization showed two major blockages that were opened by a stent procedure. He now took several new medications.

"Yeah, this is the best I've felt in years," Doug said as he sat perfectly straight in the cloth chair, a broad smile revealing deep wrinkles around his eyes and across his forehead. "I had no idea that I didn't have to live at fifty percent for the rest of my life."

His mechanically unclogged coronary arteries were just part of the equation. He'd also stopped smoking cigarettes, something that, other than a few weeks here and there, he'd done for over forty-five years. He'd also cut back from three brandies each night down to one. Like many patients who suffer a heart attack or get diagnosed with cancer, he'd begun making changes neither he nor those close to him ever thought possible.

"Physically, it sounds like you're a lot better," I said. "How about the mental side?"

"Guess you have to ask me that in a shrink's office, right?"

We both smiled. He told me that he'd been scared at first, before the catheterization and stent procedure. He started having nightmares again about his combat stint in Vietnam, something that hadn't occurred in years. But within days of leaving the hospital, he began feeling better quickly. Still, both he and the cardiologists agreed he should continue his antidepressant medication without modification. They told him that many patients had worse moods after heart procedures and that it was better to stay the course.

When Doug left my office, my biggest worry was that with time, old patterns might resurface or new unhealthy ones might spring forth. Maybe he wouldn't return to smoking or escalate his daily alcohol use again but he might start bingeing on snack foods that packed on pounds, something I'd seen with many patients over the years. Instead, Doug returned two months later looking slimmer, and our conversation prompted me to modify how I talked with patients moving forward.

"I started this Mediterranean diet," he told me.

By then, I'd heard a fair amount about the diet on TV medical segments and doctor shows with proclamations about how it reduced heart disease and made people live longer. More fruits and vegetables, more beans, peas, and nuts, less red meat and processed foods, and so forth. I told him that his cardiologist and primary care doctor would be happy to hear this, and I congratulated him on making these dietary changes. His reply caught me off guard.

"I really think it's making me feel better mentally. That's what I'm noticing most."

I didn't know how to respond. Placebo effect, right? The idea that he was doing something he believed would help his health had the self-fulfilling prophecy of doing so. But if the Mediterranean diet, and others like it, were known to improve the physical body, why was it so hard to imagine them helping the emotional mind too? For years, I'd only talked about food with people in terms of how it impacted their diabetes or high blood pressure. In psychiatry, it wasn't a priority. Not at all. But how could we argue that mental illness had biological components and not bother to ask our patients about nutrition? It didn't make any more sense than a medical or surgical provider completely avoiding the emotional impact a physical illness had on their patient. We'd all fallen into the false body-versus-mind trap. In that moment, I got a new view of our long-standing folly.

Doug continued to do well. He'd joined a veterans group and began to see himself as a mentor to others trying to lead healthier lives. After a year or so, he told me it was time to say goodbye: "There are other people who need to see you more than I do. I'm taking up a slot. Hopefully, you can make their lives better too."

I thought about how we'd gotten started and everything that led up to that moment. A medical device assessed electrical activity in his heart. The blips on the paper looked abnormal, so I drove to see his primary care doctor, Dr. Cohen, whom I'd known for years and had once worked with in the same office. Together, we reviewed this ECG, compared it to a previous one, and immediately decided he needed to see a cardiologist. Without our prior relationship, my message to Dr. Cohen would

have been sent through cluttered electronic communication. Could that
have delayed Doug's diagnosis and ultimate treatment? I'd seen it happen in other situations.

"I'm glad you're feeling so much better," I said.

He smiled. "I never thought a shrink could save your life. Man, you
just never know."

Diagnosing Doug's heart problem led him to stop smoking, drink
less, and eat better. These changes then boosted him psychologically, in
terms of how he coped with his experiences from Vietnam and saw himself in the present. Tending to the body had helped heal his mind. With
Willie, this process had worked in reverse. Unburdening his mind from
despair and suicidality had enabled him to tend to his body; he started
playing doubles tennis a few days each week with other retired men and
joined a senior fitness class.

Body and mind. Mind and body. For far too long, we've drawn a sharp
line between them. For patients, it often means seeing your general medicine or specialty doctor in one part of town and your psychiatrist or psychologist in an entirely different area. Or visiting the "medical" doctor
on the first floor of a hospital or medical office and the "mental" doctor
in the basement. For physicians, this separation has conditioned us to
believe that "body" medicine is objective and clear-cut, while "mind"
medicine is make-believe and less valuable.

But as Doug, Willie, and so many others continue to show me each
day I enter a hospital or clinic, there can never be a clean divide between
our physical and emotional selves, any more than we can live without a
functioning brain and a beating heart. These and other essential organs
all inhabit one body that works in concert to experience all the joys and
pains, all the triumphs and tragedies of this thing we call human life. The
more we can embrace this ethos as we enact laws, build hospitals, devise
health systems, and educate the array of future health care workers who
will one day face us and our loved ones in our greatest hours of need, the
better off we will all be.

ACKNOWLEDGMENTS

It's been nearly a decade since my first book was published, and for much of that time, I came to accept that I would never write another one. But in the spring of 2021, as a seventeen-student class of second-year Duke medical students shared their hospital and clinic experiences with me, the idea for this project was born. Many of the doctors they worked under seemed ill-suited to address the emotional needs of the patients who came to them, they told me. But why? During these searing conversations, I reflected on my own medical journey, and within a few weeks of that course ending, I typed the first words of this book.

It's often said that you can't go home again, but on the writing side, I feel that is exactly what I did. Jane Harrigan, freelance editor extraordinaire, once more helped me shape a series of badly disjointed thoughts into a far more cohesive outline and narrative. From there, literary agent Rebecca Gradinger took the mantle and expanded my vision of the book's potential scope. This led back to my editor, Anna deVries, who again pushed me to dig deeper to examine my motivations and insights. I can't imagine an author having a better trio of writing support. To have this twice feels like an embarrassment of riches. I must also extend thanks to other members of the publishing team, including Laura Clark, Martin

Quinn, Gabrielle Gantz, Jamilah Horton, Susannah Noel, Sara Robb with ScriptAcuity Studio, and Devereux Chatillon.

This book aims to expand beyond my own experiences and reflections, and to the extent that I've succeeded with that goal, several people deserve credit. Caroline Elton, Diana McNeill, and Aimee Zaas helped me better understand the landscape of physician well-being. Christine Wilder, Joseph Lee, Dana Clifton, and Noel Ivey are all leaders, in different ways, in the realm of addiction medicine, and the general public—and this book—are the better for their efforts. Frank deGruy, Parinda Khatri, Jürgen Unützer, and Alexander Blount each generously shared their time and insights with me from their decades-long careers working at the forefront of efforts to integrate behavioral health and primary care.

Five fellow physicians deserve special mention. Not only did Louise Aronson, Jeff Drayer, Tom Linden, Dinah Miller, and Danielle Ofri all read portions of the manuscript and provide valuable input, but their examples as physician-writers have been inspiring throughout my own career. Other physicians who offered helpful feedback include Dan Blazer II, Harvey Cohen, Jane Deveau, Warren Kinghorn, Brian Quaranta, Jattu Senesie, and Colin Smith.

My colleagues at the Durham VA Health Care System have been incredibly supportive of my career as a psychiatrist. Cindy Greenlee and Jonathan Leinbach have been most instrumental in enabling me to balance my many roles, but I am indebted to the rest of you too, even though there is not enough space to name everyone individually. We have worked hard under difficult circumstances to provide emotional care and support for our nation's military veterans, many of whom have seen both the best and worst that this world offers.

At Duke University School of Medicine, I am grateful to my colleagues in the psychiatry department—Moira Rynn, Shelley Holmer, Heather Vestal, and the many others with whom I've discussed the topics in this book over the years. Jane Gagliardi, who started at Duke Med two years before me, and who has been both an invaluable peer and mentor since, deserves special mention. Thanks also to Jeff Baker and the team at the

Trent Center for Bioethics, Humanities, and History of Medicine, for inviting me into a home of like-minded physician-scholars.

No book about a doctor's career such as mine would be possible without the patients and their family members whose well-being remains the core purpose behind everything I've written. Collectively, you have made me a better person, humbler and less selfish, and I can only continue to hope that I've returned some small part of that goodwill back into your lives over the years.

Finally, writing a book takes endless hours away from those closest to you, and for me, that will always mean my immediate family. I'll never be able to repay my gratitude for being raised by two loving parents along with an older brother who led by shining example. Calvin, Harriet, and Bryan Tweedy, your names deserve to be in print every bit as much as mine. My greatest wish is that the life I've carved out with my wife, Kerrie, mom and doctor extraordinaire, will offer that same environment of love and support for our two boys, Justin and Julian. Love always.

NOTES

INTRODUCTION

3   *most shooting deaths*: In 2021, the most recent year with available data, suicide accounted for 54 percent of all gun-related deaths (26,328 of 48,830). This percentage was nearly identical in 2020. In the years 2017–2019, suicides accounted for between 60 and 61 percent of said deaths each year. See Centers for Disease Control and Prevention, National Center for Health Statistics, https://www.cdc.gov/nchs/fastats/default.htm. Multiple Cause of Death 2021 on CDC WONDER Online Database as compiled from data provided by the fifty-seven vital statistics jurisdictions through the Vital Statistics Cooperative Program, accessed at "About Multiple Cause of Death, 1999–2020," CDC WONDER, http://wonder.cdc.gov/mcd-icd10.html.

3   *Especially in older men*: In the US, men consistently die from suicide each year at a rate about four times that of women. Men over age seventy-five have the highest risk of suicide of all groups. See "Suicide," National Institute of Mental Health, https://www.nimh.nih.gov/health/statistics/suicide.

7   *That leads critics of our field*: Criticism of psychiatry and psychiatrists spans across many medical and social science disciplines and includes several organizations, perhaps most notably the Church of Scientology, whose founder, L. Ron Hubbard, likened psychiatrists to terrorists. This article discusses some of the group's beliefs as they relate to psychiatry: Katharine Mieszkowski, "Scientology's War on Psychiatry," Salon, July 1, 2005, https://www.salon.com/2005/07/01/sci_psy/.

8   *Each year for decades*: See David Brown, "At Psychiatry Meeting, Ex-Patients Protest Psychiatric Treatment," *Washington Post*, May 4, 1992. See also Dinah Miller, "Responding to Antipsychiatry Protestors," *Clinical Psychiatry News*, August 16, 2013, https://www.mdedge.com/psychiatry

/article/77147/schizophrenia-other-psychotic-disorders/responding
-antipsychiatry.

8   *Most opposition these days*: Perhaps the most prominent source is the website Mad in America, led by journalist Robert Whitaker, the author of
several books highly critical of modern psychiatry.

8   *whose numbers have skyrocketed*: See Emily Terlizzi and Jeannine Schil-
ler, Centers for Disease Control National Center for Health Statistics,
Data Brief No. 444, September 2022, https://www.cdc.gov/nchs/products
/databriefs/db444.htm.

10 *National Institute of Mental Health (NIMH) estimates*: "2021 National Survey of Drug Use and Health (NSDUH) Releases," SAMHSA, https://
www.samhsa.gov/data/release/2021-national-survey-drug-use-and-health
-nsduh-releases.

10 *around 5 percent per year*: "2021 National Survey," SAMHSA.

10 *Suicide is consistently near the top-ten*: In 2021, suicide claimed forty-eight
thousand lives and was the eleventh leading cause of death. See "Suicide and Self Injury," Centers for Disease Control, National Center for
Health Statistics, https://www.cdc.gov/nchs/fastats/suicide.htm.

10 *Over the past two decades*: Centers for Disease Control, *Morbidity and Mortality Weekly Report*, June 8, 2018, https://www.cdc.gov/mmwr/volumes
/67/wr/pdfs/mm6722a1-H.pdf.

10 *Alcohol, tobacco, and other drugs*: See "Alcohol, Tobacco, and Other Drugs,"
SAMHSA, https://www.samhsa.gov/find-help/atod.

10 *In 2019, the National Institute on Alcohol*: "Key Substance Use and Mental
Health Indicators in the United States: Results from the 2019 National
Survey on Drug Use and Health," SAMHSA, HHS Publication No.
PEP20–07–01–001, NSDUH Series H-55, https://www.samhsa.gov/data
/sites/default/files/reports/rpt29393/2019NSDUHFFRPDFWHTML
/2019NSDUHFFR090120.htm.

10 *And the past decade has brought*: Most American news outlets have covered
the opioid epidemic repeatedly. For book-length treatments, see: Sam
Quinones, *Dreamland* (New York: Bloomsbury, 2015), and Beth Macy,
Dopesick (New York: Little, Brown, 2018).

11 *The net effect is that too many*: See Pete Earley, *Crazy* (New York: Putnam
Adult, 2006), and Christine Montross, *Waiting for an Echo* (New York:
Penguin, 2020).

11 *Medical students and young residents*: See Lisa Rotenstein, Marco Ramos,
Matthew Torre, et al., "Prevalence of Depression, Depressive Symptoms,
and Suicidal Ideation among Medical Students," *Journal of the American
Medical Association* 316, no. 21 (2016): 2214–36. See also Douglas Mata,
Marco Ramos, Narinder Bansal, et al., "Prevalence of Depression and
Depressive Symptoms among Resident Physicians," *Journal of the Amer-
ican Medical Association* 314, no. 22 (2015): 2373–83.

11 *Alcohol and drug use is also prevalent*: Michael Oreskovich, Tait Shanafelt,
Lotte Dyrbye, et al., "The Prevalence of Substance Use Disorders in

American Physicians," *American Journal of Addictions* 24, no. 1 (2015): 30–38.

11 *The rate of suicide among physicians*: See "10 Facts about Physician Suicide and Mental Health," American Foundation for Suicide Prevention, https://www.acgme.org/globalassets/PDFs/ten-facts-about-physician-suicide.pdf.

12 *Rates of anxiety and depression disorders*: Nirmita Panchal, Heather Saunders, Robin Rudowitz, and Cynthia Cox, "The Implications of COVID-19 for Mental Health and Substance Use," Kaiser Family Foundation, https://www.kff.org/coronavirus-covid-19/issue-brief/the-implications-of-covid-19-for-mental-health-and-substance-use/.

12 *Intimate partner violence rates rose*: "Impact Report: COVID-19 and Domestic Violence Trends," Council on Criminal Justice, February 23, 2021, https://counciloncj.org/impact-report-covid-19-and-domestic-violence-trends/.

I. MISEDUCATION

17 *assigned to a state-run psychiatric hospital*: All states oversee inpatient psychiatric units, most operating within specialty state psychiatric hospitals. States vary considerably as to whether to use the beds for short-term, intermediate, or long-term care. During my medical school years, North Carolina operated four such facilities; that has since been reduced to three hospitals.

26 *psychiatrists had played an important role*: Many of the forced sterilizations of this period were done on people housed in psychiatric institutions. Harvard history professor Anne Harrington devotes several pages to this past in her sweeping history of psychiatry. Anne Harrington, *Mind Fixers* (New York: W. W. Norton, 2019).

29 *At every US medical school*: The Association of American Medical Colleges (AAMC) represents US medical schools and teaching hospitals and is a go-to on most topics relevant to medical education. Data on medical school clerkship requirements is found here: "Clerkship Requirements by Discipline," Association of American Colleges, https://www.aamc.org/data-reports/curriculum-reports/data/clerkship-requirements-discipline.

29 *95 percent of medical students*: In 2011, 4 percent of medical students matched into psychiatry. While psychiatry has become a more popular career choice among medical students over the past decade (in 2022, 6 percent of medical school graduates matched in the field), more than 90 percent of medical school graduates still choose other disciplines. Mark Moran, "Psychiatry Match Numbers Increase for 11th Straight Year," Psychiatry Online, April 23, 2022, https://psychnews.psychiatryonline.org/doi/10.1176/appi.pn.2022.05.5.24?cookieSet=1.

29 *Major depression is about twenty times*: The National Institute of Mental Health (NIMH) estimates that 8.5 percent of US adults have had a

major depressive episode. In contrast, the prevalence of schizophrenia is about 0.5 percent. "Statistics," National Institute of Mental Health, https://www.nimh.nih.gov/health/statistics.

29 *Anxiety disorders, which include panic disorder*: The NIMH estimates nearly 20 percent of adults have an anxiety disorder in any given year compared with less than 3 percent with bipolar disorder. "Statistics," National Institute of Mental Health.

33 *According to a 2014 report*: "QuickStats: Percentage of Mental Health–Related* Primary Care† Office Visits, by Age Group—National Ambulatory Medical Care Survey, United States, 2010," Centers for Disease Control, *Morbidity and Mortality Weekly Report*, November 28, 2014, https://www.cdc.gov/mmwr/preview/mmwrhtml/mm6347a6.htm.

35 *Hundreds of scientific articles*: For a classic article that guided much of my third-year research efforts under the direction of Dr. James Blumenthal, see Alan Rozanski et al., "Mental Stress and the Induction of Silent Myocardial Ischemia in Patients with Coronary Artery Disease," *New England Journal of Medicine* 318 (1988): 1005–12.

35 *learning how different nondrug interventions*: Examples include dietary interventions, such as the DASH diet, aerobic exercise, and brief stress management classes, all of which reduced blood pressure in study participants with hypertension.

37 *Michelle was taking a drug*: Before the advent of the SSRI medications in the late 1980s, tricyclic antidepressants (TCAs) were the pharmacological mainstay to treat depression. They have largely fallen out of favor as a depression treatment due to a host of side effects common with higher doses needed to treat depression. Nowadays, they are more likely to be used in lower doses to treat headaches, chronic pain, and insomnia. Common TCAs include amitriptyline (Elavil), nortriptyline (Pamelor), and imipramine (Tofranil), which was one of the first drugs marketed as an antidepressant (circa mid-1950s), and the oldest antidepressant drug still in use.

2. DISSONANCE

41 *religious persecutions of the Middle Ages*: For a brief summary, see Allen Frances, *Saving Normal* (New York: Mariner, 2013).

41 *asylums of the seventeenth and eighteenth centuries*: For a brief sweep, see Ron Powers, *No One Cares about Crazy People* (New York: Hachette Books, 2017). For a deeper dive, see Roy Richard Grinker, *Nobody's Normal* (New York: W. W. Norton, 2021).

41 *gave us eugenics and lobotomies*: Anne Harrington, *Mind Fixers* (New York: W. W. Norton, 2019); Jeffrey Lieberman, *Shrinks* (New York: Little, Brown Spark, 2015).

42 *Strong Black Woman archetype*: There has been much written about this subject in the popular press, ranging from discussions of widely known

women such as Michelle Obama, Oprah Winfrey, and Serena Williams, to portrayals of black women in movies such as *Hidden Figures* and *The Color Purple*. This topic has also been the subject of many academic papers; for example, see Natalie Watson and Carla Hunter, "Anxiety and Depression among African-American Women: The Costs of Strengths and Negative Attitudes toward Psychological Help-Seeking," *Cultural Diversity and Ethnic Minority Psychology* 21, no. 4 (2015): 604–12.

44   *few exotic illnesses*: At an academic hospital like Duke, we were more likely to see people with "medical zebra" conditions, such as hemochromatosis, pheochromocytoma, and acute intermittent porphyria, for example, than at a general hospital.

45   *racist, sexist, and homophobic things*: Where should I begin? Let's go with the extreme examples. I once heard a physician, with a straight face, ask a Muslim medical student if he was a terrorist. Another time, a senior doctor told a small group of junior doctors that women shouldn't go into medicine if they wanted to have children. And off-color jokes about members of the LGBTQ community were still largely acceptable then.

56   *trainees are prone to develop*: see Paul Salkovskis and Oliver Howes, "Health Anxiety in Medical Students," *Lancet* 351, no. 9112 (1998): 1332.

57   *We didn't know about exceptional people*: See Elyn Saks, *The Center Cannot Hold* (New York: Hachette Books, 2007). The book describes her remarkable academic and personal success while living with schizophrenia. Saks also has a 2012 TED Talk with nearly five million views. See Kay Redfield Jamison, *An Unquiet Mind* (New York: Knopf, 1995). Jamison is a psychologist and prolific author of many books about mental illness, specifically bipolar disorder, which is the illness she describes living with in her memoir.

57   *Nor did we know about the everyday person*: The structure of our training in psychiatric hospitals and medical floors rather than in clinics or community nonmedical settings conditioned us to see these illnesses through the most severely disabling lenses.

3. PROXIMITY

75   *Neuroleptic malignant syndrome*: See Jeffrey Strawn, Paul Keck, and Stanley Caroff, "Neuroleptic Malignant Syndrome," *American Journal of Psychiatry* 164, no. 6 (2007): 870–76.

75   *This antiquated system remained*: This 2013 article from Johns Hopkins researchers illustrates the pitfalls (in particular, medication errors) of fully restricting psychiatric records from nonpsychiatrist doctors. Dana Kozubal et al., "Separate May Not Be Equal: A Preliminary Investigation of Clinical Correlates of Electronic Psychiatric Record Accessibility in Academic Medical Centers," *International Journal of Medical Informatics* 82, no. 4 (2013): 260–67. The current system at the hospitals where I work,

and in many other places, now allow nonpsychiatrist doctors greater access.

75   *serotonin syndrome*: See Edward Boyer and Michael Shannon, "The Serotonin Syndrome," *New England Journal of Medicine* 352 (2005): 1112–20.

76   *catatonia, a condition of unknown cause*: See Amber Edinoff et al., "Catatonia: Clinical Overview of the Diagnosis, Treatment, and Clinical Challenges," *Neurology International* 13, no. 4 (2021): 570–86.

79   *Catatonia can in some cases progress*: Julia Park et al., "Malignant Catatonia Warrants Early Psychiatric-Critical Care Collaborative Management: Two Cases and Literature Review," *Case Reports in Critical Care* 2017, article ID: 1951965, https://doi.org/10.1155/2017/1951965.

81   *While the COVID-19 pandemic has brought*: The 2020 death of ER physician Dr. Lorna Breen from suicide during the early months of the COVID-19 pandemic brought dramatic attention to the mental health needs of medical providers, including several articles in the *New York Times* among other national coverage. In 2022, Congress passed the Dr. Lorna Breen Health Care Provider Protection Act, which was signed into law by President Biden.

87   *medical procedure called a* paracentesis: For a straightforward overview of the procedure, please see Elisa M. Aponte, Shravan Katta, and Maria C. O'Rourke, "Paracentesis," National Center for Biotechnology Information, updated May 21, 2023, https://www.ncbi.nlm.nih.gov/books/NBK435998/.

91   *author of the 2018 book*: See Caroline Elton, *Also Human: The Inner Lives of Doctors* (New York: Basic Books, 2018).

91   *more likely to misuse prescription sedatives*: See Lisa Merlo and Mark Gold, "Prescription Opioid Abuse and Dependence among Physicians: Hypotheses and Treatment," *Harvard Review of Psychiatry* 16, no. 3 (2008): 181–94.

91   *doctors consistently have suicide rates*: It is estimated that between three hundred and four hundred US physicians die from suicide each year and that the suicide rate among physicians doubles that in the general population. For an article on the subject published during the time that I was training, see Eva Schernhammer, "Taking Their Own Lives—the High Rate of Physician Suicide," *New England Journal of Medicine* 352 (2005): 2473–76, https://www.nejm.org/doi/full/10.1056/nejmp058014.

92   *might go into one's permanent record*: For decades, physicians renewing or seeking a medical license were asked questions about whether they had received mental health care. Many feel that this discouraged physicians from treatment. For a thoughtful perspective on the culture of medicine and barriers to seeking mental health services among doctors, see Seema Jilani, "Why So Many Doctors Treat Their Mental Health in Secret," *New York Times*, March 30, 2022.

94   *Black residents are more likely*: See Usha Lee McFarling, "Black Doctors

Are Forced Out of Training Programs at Far Higher Rates than White Residents," STAT, June 20, 2022.

98   *Dr. Elton, and others*: See Elton, *Also Human*; Jilani, "Why So Many Doctors."

4. SEPARATE AND UNEQUAL

103   *it wasn't like this everywhere*: In speaking with psychiatrists who trained in Maryland, Massachusetts, New York, and Pennsylvania either before or during the same time as I did, I learned that each of these states used an ambulance as the primary means of transport from an emergency room to a freestanding psychiatric hospital. According to them, the same held true for colleagues who trained in nearby states.

105   *psychiatric hospitalizations peaked*: J. Sanbourne Bockoven, *Moral Treatment in Community Mental Health* (New York: Springer, 1972).

106   *psychiatric hospital deinstitutionalization movements*: There have been many accounts that describe this pivotal era in the history of American psychiatry. For a thorough yet concise recent summary, see Thomas Insel, *Healing: Our Path from Mental Illness to Mental Health* (New York: Penguin, 2022).

108   *the more lethal options of guns*: Konstantinos Tsirigotis, Wojciech Gruszczynski, and Marta Tsirigotis, "Gender Differentiation in Methods of Suicide Attempts," *Medical Science Monitor* 17, no. 8 (2011): 65–70.

111   *how common it was for people*: It is difficult to find US data on this, but many ER medical providers see this daily. Interestingly, academic data in this area mainly comes from Canada, where researchers have published many articles on the topic. For example, see Natasha Saunders et al., "Use of the Emergency Department as a First Point of Contact for Mental Health Care by Immigrant Youth in Canada: A Population-Based Study," *Canadian Medical Association Journal* 190, no. 40 (2018): 1183–91. These authors found that 60 percent of immigrant youth, generally poorer than native residents, received their first mental health care in the ER. One imagines that in the US health care system, where health insurance access is more limited than in Canada, those numbers could possibly be higher for age-matched controls.

115   *A 2016 study revealed*: Jane Zhu, Astha Singal, and Renee Hsia, "Emergency Department Length-of-Stay for Psychiatric Visits Was Significantly Longer than for Nonpsychiatric Visits, 2002–2011," *Health Affairs* 35, no. 9 (2016): 1698–706.

115   *There are far fewer psychiatric beds*: This is a complex issue to understand, but the extensive wait times in emergency rooms and the common scenario of admitting patients in psychiatric crisis to ill-equipped general medicine and pediatric floors underscores the problem. For a deep dive, please see: *The Psychiatric Bed Crisis in the US: Understanding the Problem and Moving toward Solutions* (Washington, DC: American Psychiatric

Association, 2022), https://www.psychiatry.org/getmedia/81f685f1–036e
-4311–8dfc-e13ac425380f/APA-Psychiatric-Bed-Crisis-Report-Full.pdf.

115   *likelier to lack health insurance*: Kathleen Rowan, Donna McAlpine, and
Lynn Blewett, "Access and Cost Barriers to Mental Health Care by Insurance Status, 1999 to 2010," *Health Affairs* 32, no. 10 (2013): 1723–30.

115   *those insured disproportionately*: Rowan, McAlpine, and Blewett, "Access
and Cost Barriers."

115   *psychiatry doesn't pay*: For an example of how this unfolds in our nation's
most populous state, see Paul Sisson, "Hospitals Lose Money Caring for
Mental Health Patients: Is There a Better Way?," *San Diego Union Tri-
bune*, July 1, 2019.

116   *nearly one in six adults*: See "Health Insurance Coverage of the Total Population," Kaiser Family Foundation, State Health Facts, https://www
.kff.org/other/state-indicator/total-population/?currentTimeframe=12
&sortModel=%7B%22colId%22:%22Location%22,%22sort%22:%22
asc%22%7D. The database covers the years 2008 (prior to the 2010 passage of the ACA) up through 2021.

126   *Psychiatry beds, in contrast to medical*: For a clear explanation of this, see
Insel, *Healing*.

126   *Between 2005 and 2010*: Samantha Raphelson, "How the Loss of US
Psychiatric Hospitals Led to a Mental Health Crisis," NPR, November
30, 2017, https://www.npr.org/2017/11/30/567477160/how-the-loss-of
-u-s-psychiatric-hospitals-led-to-a-mental-health-crisis.

127   *By law, in North Carolina*: Taylor Knopf, "More NC Psych Patients Are
Ending Up Handcuffed in a Police Car. Why?," North Carolina Health
News, December 14, 2020, https://www.northcarolinahealthnews.org
/2020/12/14/more-nc-psych-patients-are-ending-up-handcuffed-in-a
-police-car-why/.

127   *prolific author on psychiatric issues*: Dr. Miller wrote the popular blog *Shrink
Rap* for over ten years as well as coauthoring a book of the same name;
see Dinah Miller, Annette Hanson, and Steven Daviss, *Shrink Rap: Three
Psychiatrists Explain Their Work* (Baltimore: Johns Hopkins University
Press, 2011).

127   *In 2016, Miller, along with psychiatrist colleague*: Dinah Miller and Annette Hanson, *Committed: The Battle over Psychiatric Involuntary Care*
(Baltimore: Johns Hopkins University Press, 2016).

128   *treating mental illness is a bipartisan issue*: Examples include the 21st Century Cures Act that was signed into law by President Barack Obama in
2016, and the STOP Act signed by North Carolina governor Roy Cooper
in 2017. Both passed legislatively with overwhelming bipartisan support.

128   *North Carolina legislators passed a law*: Taylor Knopf, "Despite Pitfalls,
Counties Leave Psych Patient Transport in Sheriffs' Hands," North Carolina Health News, March 23, 2021, https://www.northcarolinahealthnews
.org/2021/03/23/psychiatric-patient-involuntary-commitment-transport
-in-sheriffs-hands/.

128   *North Carolina became the fortieth state*: See "Governor Cooper Signs Medicaid Expansion into Law," North Carolina Office of the Governor, March 27, 2023, https://governor.nc.gov/news/press-releases/2023 /03/27/governor-cooper-signs-medicaid-expansion-law.

5. ON PILLS AND NEEDLES

135   *at the time a radical proposal*: Official remarks from Dr. James Campbell in his then-role as president of the American Pain Society, November 11, 1996. Colin Fernandes, "The Fifth Vital Sign," *Federal Practitioner*, December 2010, https://cdn.mdedge.com/files/s3fs-public/Document /September-2017/027120026.pdf

136   *influential national health organizations*: This included the Veterans Health Administration (VHA) and The Joint Commission (formerly JCHAO).

136   *entered the market in 1996*: Several books and news accounts have told the story of Purdue Pharmaceuticals and OxyContin. For example, see Haider Warraich, *The Song of Our Scars* (New York: Basic Books, 2022). See also Anna Lembke, *Drug Dealer, MD* (Baltimore: Johns Hopkins University Press, 2016).

138   *given the widespread societal stigma*: For a summary, see Lawrence Yang et al., "Stigma and Substance Use Disorders: An International Phenomenon," *Current Opinion in Psychiatry* 30, no. 5 (2017): 378–88.

140   *despite women entering the military*: In 2008, a few years after I met Natalie, women comprised between 10 and 20 percent of active duty service members across the five service branches. "Demographic Profile of the Active-Duty Enlisted Force," Military Leadership Diversity Commission, issue paper #19, March 2010, https://diversity.defense.gov/Portals/51 /Documents/Resources/Commission/docs/Issue%20Papers/Paper%20 19%20-%20Demographics%20of%20Active%20Duty%20Enlisted.pdf.

149   *Media coverage was equally enthusiastic*: Howard Markel, "For Addicts, Relief May Be an Office Visit Away," *New York Times*, October 27, 2002.

150   *8 percent of eligible physicians*: Emma McGinty et al., "Medication for Opioid Use Disorder: A National Survey of Primary Care Physicians," *Annals of Internal Medicine* 173, no. 2 (2021): 160–62.

151   *US overdose deaths related to opioids*: "Drug Overdose Death Rates," National Institute on Drug Abuse, https://nida.nih.gov/research-topics/trends -statistics/overdose-death-rates.

151   *In 2021, opioid-related deaths*: "Drug Overdose Death Rates," National Institute on Drug Abuse.

151   *Preliminary data suggests these rates*: "Provisional Drug Overdose Death Counts," Centers for Disease Control and Prevention, National Center for Health Statistics, National Vital Statistics System, https://www.cdc .gov/nchs/nvss/vsrr/drug-overdose-data.htm.

157   *women were far more likely than men*: Some researchers assert this is a function of gender sampling bias, meaning that women with these

behavioral and emotional characteristics are more likely to present to traditional mental health treatment settings whereas men are more likely to be seen in substance-related treatment settings or in jail/prison settings. They call this *sampling bias*. See Randy Sansone and Lisa Sansone, "Gender Patterns in Borderline Personality Disorder," *Innovations in Clinical Neuroscience* 8, no. 5 (2011): 16–20.

157 *a label whose stigma within psychiatry*: In similar fashion to people who misuse drugs, those with borderline personality disorder are often seen as being deliberately self-destructive and harmful to other people. For a classic Hollywood depiction, consider the character played by Glenn Close in the 1987 thriller *Fatal Attraction*. For a recent article on this stigma, see Susan Krauss Whitbourne, "Why People with Borderline Personality Disorder Are Treated So Poorly, and the Difference Greater Empathy Could Make," *Psychology Today*, January 29, 2022.

160 *she'd also get a take-home Narcan*: This medication is an opioid antagonist that rapidly reverses an overdose. Increasingly, emergency departments across the US have begun implementing programs to distribute the drug in this setting. Data is still being collected on its effectiveness. For example, Alexander Gunn et al., "The Emergency Department as an Opportunity for Naloxone Distribution," *Western Journal of Emergency Medicine* 19, no. 6 (2018): 1036–42. See also Aaron Dora-Laskey, "Piloting a Statewide Emergency Department Take-Home Naloxone Program: Improving the Quality of Care for Patients at Risk of Opioid Overdose," *Academic Emergency Medicine* 29, no. 4 (2022): 442–55.

160 *test strips to help her avoid fentanyl*: Fentanyl is about fifty times more potent than heroin and one hundred times more so than morphine. Powdered fentanyl is often mixed with heroin, cocaine, and amphetamines and made into pills that look similar to other prescription opioids. Many people may be unaware that their drugs are laced with fentanyl. Providing fentanyl test strips is a harm-reduction strategy. See Rafael Lima et al., "Feasibility of Emergency Department-Based Fentanyl Test Strip Distribution," *Journal of Addiction Medicine* 16, no. 6 (2022): 730–32.

160 *emergency rooms are also nowadays better equipped*: See Ian Reynolds and Victoria Yastishock, "Emergency Departments Can Help People with Opioid Use Disorder Start Treatment," Pew, May 18, 2021, https://www .pewtrusts.org/en/research-and-analysis/articles/2021/05/18/emergency -departments-can-help-people-with-opioid-use-disorder-start-treatment.

160 *Or did she die from an overdose*: "Understanding the Opioid Overdose Epidemic," Centers for Disease Control and Prevention, https://www.cdc .gov/opioids/basics/epidemic.html.

6. FROM HEAD TO TOE

165 *A widely discussed 2006 report*: Craig Colton and Ronald Manderscheid, "Congruencies in Increased Mortality Rates, Years of Potential Life

Lost, and Causes of Death among Public Mental Health Clients in Eight States," *Preventing Chronic Disease* 3, no. 2 (2006): 1–14.

165 *People with psychiatric disorders*: For example, see M. Robin DiMatteo, Heidi Lepper, and Thomas Croghan, "Depression Is a Risk Factor for Noncompliance with Medical Treatment," *Archives of Internal Medicine* 160 (2000): 2101–7.

165 *They are likelier to misuse substances*: Substance misuse is a mental health problem in and of itself and is often comorbid with other mental illnesses.

165 *have less nutritious diets*: DiMatteo, Lepper, and Croghan, "Depression Is a Risk Factor."

165 *Their sleep patterns are often highly irregular*: Sleep disturbances are part of the diagnostic criteria for bipolar disorder and major depressive disorder, and also are common in people with anxiety disorders and psychotic disorders.

165 *could cause significant weight gain*: For a general overview, see Victor Mazereel et al., "Impact of Psychotropic Medication Effects on Obesity and the Metabolic Syndrome in People with Serious Mental Illness," *Frontiers in Endocrinology* 11 (2020): 1–10.

166 *Millions of people come to hospitals*: Judd Hollander and Maureen Chase, "Evaluation of the Adult with Chest Pain in the Emergency Department," UpToDate, updated on September 21, 2022, https://www.uptodate .com/contents/evaluation-of-the-adult-with-chest-pain-in-the-emergency -department. There are over seven million ER visits each year in the US related to chest pain, ranking it near the top of all causes.

166 *a sizable number*: More than three-quarters of people who come to emergency departments with chest pain do not have a cardiac or respiratory emergency. As many as half are thought to be due to anxiety. See Guillaume Foldes-Busque et al., "A Closer Look at the Relationships between Panic Attacks, Emergency Department Visits and Non-Cardiac Chest Pain," *Journal of Health Psychology* 24, no. 6 (2019): 717–25.

171 *I was just beginning to understand*: This problem has only worsened in the intervening years, especially in the aftermath of the COVID-19 pandemic. For a recent analysis, see Hemangi Modi, Kendal Orgera, and Atul Grover, "Exploring Barriers to Mental Health Care in the US," *Association of American Medical Colleges (AAMC) Issue Brief*, October 10, 2022.

177 *much of what doctors hear*: For a thoughtful discussion about the subject, please see chapter 5 in Atul Gawande, *Better* (New York: Henry Holt, 2006).

178 *most juries sided with doctors*: See Philip Peters, "Twenty Years of Evidence on the Outcomes of Malpractice Claims," *Clinical Orthopedics and Related Research* 467, no. 2 (2009): 352–57.

178 *overwhelming majority of claims*: Peters, "Twenty Years of Evidence."

182 *black women are about three times*: Peter Izmirly et al., "Prevalence of Systemic Lupus Erythematosus in the United States: Estimates from a

Meta-Analysis of the Centers for Disease Control and Prevention National Lupus Registries," *Arthritis & Rheumatology* 73, no. 6 (2021): 991–96.

182 *"more common in blacks than in whites"*: See Damon Tweedy, *Black Man in a White Coat* (New York: Picador, 2015).

185 *It affected multiple organ systems*: Lupus, not unlike diabetes, most notoriously impacts the kidneys, but it can also cause damage to the skin, heart, lungs, joints, tendons, and brain.

185 *trained in both internal medicine and psychiatry*: The first combined psychiatry residency programs began in the late 1980s as a way to prepare doctors for integrated care. Duke's program took root in the mid-1990s, and has been led by program alumnus Dr. Jane Gagliardi for several years. As of 2019, there are fourteen combined internal medicine–psychiatry programs in the US and six combined family medicine–psychiatry programs. For further details and updates, see "Residency Programs," Association of Medicine and Psychiatry, https://assocmedpsych.org/studentstrainees/residency-programs.

186 *not in the way it was done*: Historically, health insurers have separated payment processes for mental health care and general medical care. This has certainly contributed to many of the problems we face today in terms of people being unable to readily access mental health care.

7. LOST AND FOUND

194 *Donepezil belonged to a class*: Donepezil, sold under the brand name Aricept, is a reversible acetylcholinesterase inhibitor, approved by the FDA in 1996 to slow the progression of mild dementia.

194 *A newer drug, one that worked*: Memantine, sold as Namenda, works at a different receptor system (NMDA). It was approved by the FDA in 2003 with the intent for use in moderate to severe dementia.

195 *Dementia is one of the most feared*: Donovan Maust et al., "Perception of Dementia Risk and Preventative Actions among US Adults Aged 50 to 64 Years," *JAMA Neurology* 77, no. 2 (2019): 259–62.

195 *when younger people worry*: "Perception of Aging during Each Decade of Life after Age 30," West Health Institute and NORC at the University of Chicago, Issue Brief, https://www.norc.org/PDFs/WHI-NORC-Aging-Survey/Brief_WestHealth_A_2017–03_DTPv2.pdf.

196 *It also takes an exacting toll*: Primary caretakers of people with dementia have been shown to experience challenges physically, psychologically, socially, and financially. For a review published around the time I saw Earl, see Henry Brodaty, "Family Caregivers of People with Dementia," *Dialogues in Clinical Neuroscience* 11, no. 2 (2009): 217–28.

196 *Doctors struggle when providing care*: For example, see Ladson Hinton et al., "Practice Constraints, Behavioral Problems, and Dementia Care: Primary

Care Physicians' Perspectives," *Journal of General Internal Medicine* 22, no. 11 (2007): 1487–92.

210   *a 2019 book that confronts*: Louise Aronson, *Elderhood* (New York: Blooms-bury, 2019).

211   *a movement was afoot*: For a good overview of the rationale for the Lon-gitudinal Integrated Curriculum, see Ann N. Poncelet, Karen E. Hauer, and Bridget O'Brien, "The Longitudinal Integrated Clerkship," *AMA Journal of Ethics*, November 2009.

212   *Between 2010 and 2016*: "Longitudinal Integrated Clerkships at US Med-ical Schools," Association of American Colleges, https://www.aamc.org /data-reports/curriculum-reports/data/longitudinal-integrated-clerkships -us-medical-schools.

212   *more have been established*: Close to home, Duke's LIC program began in 2017 and, starting with the 2023–24 academic year, will be incorporated in part into the full curriculum for all second-year medical students.

212   *despite the added logistical challenges*: In this educational model, students are often paired up individually with faculty in clinic settings, necessi-tating more challenging coordination than placing students in the tra-ditional hospital model. For a recent review, see Maggie Bartlett et al., "The Do's, Don'ts, and Don't Knows of Establishing a Sustainable Longitudinal Integrated Clerkship," *Perspectives on Medical Education* 9 (2020): 5–19.

8. DIAGNOSE AND TREAT

220   *effective non-medication strategies*: Examples of non-medication strate-gies include physical therapy, dietary modification, stress management groups, meditation, stretching exercises, and acupuncture, among many others.

222   *Over the past decade*: Centers for Disease Control, National Center for Health Statistics, https://www.cdc.gov/nchs/products/databriefs/db419.htm.

222   *among the most widely dispensed categories*: "National Ambulatory Medi-cal Care Survey: 2018 National Summary Tables," Centers for Disease Control, https://www.cdc.gov/nchs/data/ahcd/namcs_summary/2018 -namcs-web-tables-508.pdf.

222   *six psychiatric meds made the top-twenty-five*: These include sertraline, es-citalopram, bupropion, trazodone, dextroamphetamine, and fluoxetine. "The Top 200 of 2020," ClinCalc.com, https://clincalc.com/DrugStats /Top200Drugs.aspx.

222   *more likely to receive these drugs*: For an engaging look at this issue, see Su-zanne Koven, "Should Mental Health Be a Primary-Care Doctor's Job," *New Yorker*, October 21, 2013.

223   *rate of antidepressant use*: Laura Pratt, Debra Brody, and Quiping Gu, "Antidepressant Use in Persons Aged 12 or Older, 2005–2008," Centers

for Disease Control and Prevention, National Center of Health Statistics, https://pubmed.ncbi.nlm.nih.gov/22617183/.

223 *women took them more than twice*: Emily Terlizzi and Tina Norris, "Mental Health Treatment among Adults: United States, 2020," Centers for Disease Control, National Center for Health Statistics, https://www.cdc.gov/nchs/products/databriefs/db419.htm.

225 *Direct-to-consumer advertising*: In 1997, the Food and Drug Administration (FDA) allowed television and radio advertisements for drug manufacturers to market their products. For a brief analysis of this decision at the time, see John Schwartz, "FDA Relaxes Rules for On-Air Drug Ads," *Washington Post*, August 9, 1997. The rest, as the saying goes, is history. Before long, we were inundated with ads for cholesterol meds, allergy meds, depression meds, and, of course, erectile dysfunction drugs.

227 *a 2011* New York Times *article*: Gardiner Harris, "Talk Doesn't Pay, So Psychiatry Turns Instead to Drug Therapy," *New York Times*, March 5, 2011.

229 *our collective desire for quick fixes*: One need look no further than the latest fad promising us we'll lose "thirty pounds in thirty days."

230 *Yet only a tiny fraction*: Let's go back further. Among boys who play high school basketball, just 3.5 percent will play college basketball (and only 1 percent at the Division I level). Of this tiny fraction, 20 percent will play professional basketball, most overseas or in minor leagues in the United States. Just 1 percent of college basketball players wind up in the NBA. Lesson: hit those books!

232 *misdiagnosis is common in both directions*: For interesting dueling perspectives on the subject, see Daniel Smith, Nassir Ghaemi, and Mark Zimmerman, "Is Underdiagnosis the Main Pitfall When Diagnosing Bipolar Disorder?," *British Medical Journal* 340 (2010): 686–87.

233 *some authors exploring how the condition*: See, for example, Nassir Ghaemi, *A First-Rate Madness* (New York: Penguin, 2011). See also Kay Redfield Jamison, *Touched with Fire* (New York: Free Press, 1993).

234 *increasingly, mental health nurse practitioners*: For a deep dive into how mental health NPs are filling the psychiatric prescribing void, especially in rural and underserved areas, see Armo Cai et al., "Trends in Mental Health Care Delivery by Psychiatrists and Nurse Practitioners in Medicare, 2011 to 2019," *Health Affairs* 41, no. 9 (2022): 1222–30.

236 *the most frequently expressed*: See, for example, Gary Greenberg, *The Book of Woe* (New York: Plume, 2014), and Allen Frances, *Saving Normal* (New York: Mariner, 2014).

236 *outside of medical conditions*: There are in fact several physical conditions known to cause depression. A short, partial list includes hypothyroidism, vitamin B_{12} deficiency, lupus, multiple sclerosis, and adrenal insufficiency. Many nonpsychiatric medications can cause or worsen depression too, including some blood pressure medications, corticosteroids (used to treat many things), isotretinoin (acne medicine), and a handful of drugs

used to treat rheumatological illness. Any good medical workup needs to take these considerations into account.

236   *It is in this framework*: One can find many critiques in this vein. Examples include the Citizens Commission on Human Rights and various editorials found on the website Mad in America.

238   *numbers that define certain chronic diseases*: Throughout medical school and the early part of my career, blood pressure readings of 140/90 mmHg or greater were the criteria for diagnosing hypertension, with a value of 120/80 considered optimum, or ideal. In 2017, the American Heart Association changed the criteria to 130/80 as the hypertension cutoff with 120/80 or lower now considered "normal" rather than "ideal." The report noted that the number of people diagnosed with hypertension would triple among men under age forty-five and double among women of the same age. One year, they did not have hypertension, and the next year, they did. These determinations are based on periodic meetings of expert consensus, and we can anticipate these may change over time as more data is available. I am in no way trying to criticize their approach; rather I'm pointing out that numbers in and of themselves are not as perfect as we might view them at any point in time.

238   *Laboratory results considered normal*: When I began medical school in 1996, the most commonly used cutoff for diagnosing diabetes was a fasting blood glucose of 140 mg/dl. The following year, based on expert consensus, the number was reduced to 126 mg/dl. Since 2009, the HbA1c test, which had been available for decades, has become one of the primary ways that diabetes is now diagnosed. There is also a pre-diabetes category that previously did not exist and whose threshold is likely to shift.

238   *among the most common reasons*: Lars Stovner et al., "The Global Prevalence of Headache: An Update, with Analysis of the Influences of Methodological Factors on Prevalence Estimates," *Journal of Headache and Pain* 23 (2022): 1–17.

238   *a 2017* New Yorker *essay*: Atul Gawande, "The Heroism of Incremental Care," *New Yorker*, January 15, 2017.

239   *the same types psychiatrists used*: Common drugs used to treat headaches include the tricyclic antidepressants amitriptyline and nortriptyline, which, prior to the introduction of SSRIs, were first-line medications for depression. Some patients are also prescribed lamotrigine and valproic acid for headaches, drugs that are also commonly used for bipolar disorder.

239   *The US fares poorly*: Many writers and commentators have explored this subject. See, for example, Elisabeth Rosenthal, *An American Sickness* (New York: Penguin, 2017).

239   *one of patients' most common complaints*: I've heard many patients say this about their primary care doctors, and I imagine they've probably said that about me to other doctors. For further reading, see David Dugdale,

Ronald Epstein, and Steven Pantilat, "Time and the Physician-Patient Relationship," *Journal of General Internal Medicine* 14, suppl. 1 (1999): S34–S40.

239   *opening concierge practices*: For a personal account, see Dorothy Serna, "Lifestyle Medicine in a Concierge Practice: My Journey," *American Journal of Lifestyle Medicine* 13, no. 4 (2019): 367–70.

240   *for the last several decades*: Many authors cite Robert Spitzer's lead role with the *DSM-III* publication in 1980 with ushering in this change. The release of the SSRIs in the late 1980s and early 1990s, along with several brain research initiatives, has undoubtedly pushed us further toward "medicine" and further away from "psychology" as the fundamental underpinning of our work.

243   *all-encompassing explanations*: For a patient-friendly quick summary of various factors that contribute to higher rates of depression in women than men, see Mayo Clinic Staff, "Depression in Women: Understanding the Gender Gap," Mayo Clinic, https://www.mayoclinic.org/diseases -conditions/depression/in-depth/depression/art-20047725.

243   *In Erica's case, medication in the context*: For an engaging guide on what they describe as "a relational guide to psychopharmacology," see Warren Kinghorn and Abraham Nussbaum, *Prescribing Together* (Washington, DC: American Psychiatric Association, 2021). Another helpful book in this realm is Abraham Nussbaum, *The Finest Traditions of My Calling* (New Haven, CT: Yale University Press, 2016).

9. INTEGRATION

252   *Psychiatrists, as it turns out*: Based on data obtained in 2009 and 2010 (early in my career as a psychiatrist), psychiatrists were much less likely than other medical specialists to accept insurance. Only 55 percent accepted private insurance, compared with 89 percent among other physicians. The numbers for Medicare acceptance were nearly identical. With Medicaid, the numbers were 43 percent acceptance by psychiatrists and 73 percent among all other physicians. See Tara Bishop et al., "Acceptance of Insurance by Psychiatrists and the Implications for Access to Mental Health Care," *JAMA Psychiatry* 71, no. 2 (2014): 176–81.

253   *celebrated writer and primary care doctor*: In addition to being a prolific author of several works of nonfiction and many more essays in prestigious outlets that explore the practice of medicine across varied dimensions, Dr. Ofri is editor in chief and cofounder of the *Bellevue Literary Review* (BLR), a health-oriented literary journal.

254   *That left primary care doctors*: In a recent study, researchers found that the proportion of primary care visits that addressed mental health concerns increased from 10 percent in 2006–2007 to 15.9 percent by 2018. There is every reason to think these numbers likely have increased since. Lisa Rotenstein, Samuel Edwards, and Bruce Landon, "Adult Primary Care

Physician Visits Increasingly Address Mental Health Concerns," *Health Affairs* 42, no. 2 (2023): 163–71.

262   *From studies conducted in varied*: Much of the pioneering work in this field took place at the University of Washington School of Medicine. For an article that summarizes the history of collaborative care implementation, see Wayne Katon et al., "Collaborative Depression Care: History, Evolution and Ways to Enhance Dissemination and Sustainability," *General Hospital Psychiatry* 32, no. 5 (2010): 1–15.